Dr Paul Gow is an Australian Gastroenterologist. He completed his medical degree at Monash University and a Doctorate of Medicine through the University of Melbourne in the area of liver physiology. After completing his fellowship in Gastroenterology (specialising in gut and liver disease), he undertook two further years of specialist liver disease training in Oxford and Birmingham in the United Kingdom.

He is an Associate Professor of Medicine at the University of Melbourne. His current public practice is as senior consultant liver transplant physician with the Victorian Liver Transplant Unit based at the Austin Hospital. He has published more than 150 academic papers on the areas of liver health and disease.

Dr Gow lives in Melbourne with his wife, three children, dog, three cats and six chickens.

LIVER BETTER LIFE

Dr PAUL GOW

MACMILLAN
Pan Macmillan Australia

Pan Macmillan acknowledges the Traditional Custodians of country throughout Australia and their connections to lands, waters and communities. We pay our respect to Elders past and present and extend that respect to all Aboriginal and Torres Strait Islander peoples today. We honour more than sixty thousand years of storytelling, art and culture.

First published 2021 in Macmillan by Pan Macmillan Australia Pty Ltd
1 Market Street, Sydney, New South Wales, Australia, 2000

NATIONAL LIBRARY OF AUSTRALIA

A catalogue record for this book is available from the National Library of Australia

Typeset in 12/16pt Adobe Caslon Pro by Midland Typesetters, Australia
Printed by IVE

Figure 5.1: Mediterranean Diet Pyramid, illustration by George Middleton, reproduced with kind permission by Oldways. Figure 5.2: Graph adapted from FH Messerli, 'Chocolate consumption, cognitive function, and Nobel Laureates', *The New England Journal of Medicine*, 2012, 367(16): 1562–1564, doi:10.1056/NEJMon1211064. Figure 7.1: Graph adapted from JH O'Keefe, KA Bybee and CJ Lavie, 'Alcohol and cardiovascular health: the razor-sharp double-edged sword', *Journal of the American College of Cardiology*, 2007, 50(11):1009–1014, doi:10.1016/j.jacc.2007.04.089.

MIX
Paper from responsible sources
FSC® C018183
FSC www.fsc.org

The paper in this book is FSC® certified.
FSC® promotes environmentally responsible, socially beneficial and economically viable management of the world's forests.

To the wonder of nature and the eternal fascination of science.

Contents

Part 1

Your liver

Chapter 1

Is there fat lurking in your liver?

So, you've reached 40, and frankly, you're holding it all together pretty well. You exercise, eat reasonably well and are presentable, at least when you make the effort. But let me ask you this. Are you carrying a little extra fat around your middle? For me as a physician and liver specialist 'belly fat' is a sign that you have fatty liver disease. And we should talk.

It is normal to have some fat across the abdomen; it encases and protects the organs. However, if you have too much internal fat in your abdominal cavity – the scientific term for this fat is visceral fat – it's likely you also have microscopic droplets of fat deposited inside your liver cells. A little bit of fat in your liver is fine, but if just 5% of your liver cells have fat in them, you have a disease you may not have even heard of. That disease is fatty liver disease. Fatty liver can be caused by a number of things: excess alcohol can do it, and so can some medications, as well as viruses such as hepatitis B and C. However, the most common cause of fatty liver is the excess of the Western lifestyle. Being overweight, a poor diet and inadequate exercise all contribute to the perfect storm – fatty liver.

What's the problem? Well, excess liver fat causes damage to the liver cells. And then the cells swell and eventually die (called non-alcoholic steatohepatitis or NASH). This can lead to scarring (cirrhosis), liver cancer and liver failure. And that's just the start.

Fatty liver is the canary in the coalmine

What typically comes as a surprise to my patients is just how common fatty liver disease is. It's not just you – between one quarter and one half the population of the Western world have the condition.[1] But despite fatty liver disease being very common, the majority of people don't die as a direct consequence of it. In fact, many liver physicians reassure their patients that fatty liver disease is benign, unlikely to kill them and nothing to worry about. This reassurance is almost certainly unwarranted. If you have liver inflammation from fatty liver you should be concerned; long-term studies suggest cirrhosis may develop in up to 25% of this group and is a major cause of premature death.[2]

What's killing us?

To live long and live well are pretty standard goals most of us share. But let's look over the abyss for a moment.

The 10 most common causes of death in Australia are:

1. heart attack (ischemic heart disease)
2. dementia
3. stroke
4. lung cancer
5. emphysema
6. diabetes
7. blood and lymph cancer
8. bowel cancer
9. heart failure
10. kidney failure.

Liver disease comes in at number 13 on this list. At face value, the top 10 conditions all seem quite separate and distinct. Yet for 7 of the 10 (the exceptions are lung cancer, emphysema, and blood and lymph cancer) the driving force behind them is the same abnormal physiological mechanism. Elevated levels of insulin contribute to the development of heart disease, dementia, stroke, diabetes, bowel cancer and kidney failure. The clinical hallmark of elevated levels of insulin is fatty liver.

Insulin and the metabolic syndrome

Insulin is one of the primary hormones in the body. Its principal role is to control the levels of sugar in the blood. When you eat a meal, food is broken down and sugar is absorbed into the blood. Insulin is then released by the pancreas, facilitating the movement of sugar from the blood into the organs where it is needed. Insulin levels then fall away once this job is done. In many of us this simple mechanism is being dramatically disrupted.

Insulin resistance is one of the basic pathological process that is driving the development of fatty liver disease, heart attack, stroke, cancer, heart failure and kidney failure.

Making poor food choices, snacking, not exercising enough, gaining weight, sleeping poorly and stress all contribute to insulin levels being chronically elevated. As a result of these lifestyle factors, insulin levels are abnormally high, and fail to fall back to healthy levels between digestive cycles. The organs that take up glucose cannot cope with chronically elevated insulin levels, and respond by reducing their insulin receptors on the cells. These receptors are on every cell in the body and allow the insulin to do its job of allowing sugar into the cells. This reduction in the responsiveness of insulin receptors then sets off a vicious cycle. In this situation, insulin is still produced but the body becomes more and more resistant to its influence. Larger and larger amounts of insulin are required to exert the same influence. This syndrome is called insulin resistance.

Increased insulin production initially controls the blood sugar. As the condition progresses, however, control of blood sugar levels is lost. The medical term for this is type 2 diabetes, or maturity onset diabetes.

Although the principal role of insulin is to control blood sugar levels, chronically elevated insulin levels seen in people with insulin resistance results in widespread deleterious health consequences. Over-production of insulin directly leads to fatty liver disease. High concentrations of insulin also result in elevated levels of cholesterol and triglycerides (fats in the blood). This in turn contributes to damage to blood vessel walls in the heart, brain and kidneys; increasing the risk of heart attack, stroke and kidney failure. The insulin also impacts the blood vessel wall compliance, resulting in high blood pressure. High blood pressure acts in concert with the elevated cholesterol levels, further increasing the risk of heart attack, stroke and kidney failure. Insulin also leads to fat deposition, especially to excess visceral fat, and is one of the primary hormones involved in appetite control. Insulin drives hunger. This means that the over-production of insulin, which may have been exacerbated by excess weight, can lead to more weight gain and carries on the viscous cycle of visceral fat deposition.

The shared aetiology (insulin resistance) of excess abdominal fat, high blood pressure, high cholesterol and diabetes are very strongly linked. When a person is diagnosed with 3 or more of these conditions they have what is termed 'metabolic syndrome'.

Metabolic syndrome isn't a disease by itself, but rather a collection of conditions that commonly occur together. The syndrome is caused by insulin resistance resulting from excess visceral fat.

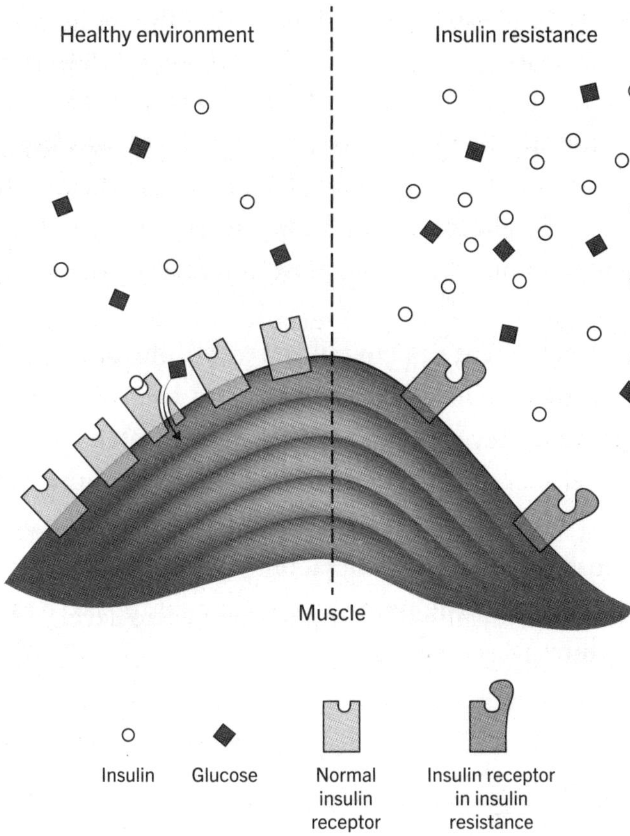

Figure 1.1 In a healthy environment (on the left) insulin molecules bind to the insulin receptor allowing easy access of glucose into the cell. When there is insulin resistance (on the right), insulin receptor numbers are reduced and the insulin receptor works inefficiently. The result is increased insulin and glucose levels in the blood.

Criteria for the diagnosis of the metabolic syndrome

1 Increased waist circumference
2 Increased triglycerides
3 Reduced HDL (good) cholesterol
4 High blood pressure
5 Diabetes

Metabolic syndrome most often occurs in people with excess abdominal fat – but a 'thick' waist is not always necessary. This syndrome is also found in people within a normal weight and waist range who are inactive or eat the wrong foods. However, excess abdominal fat is the strongest risk factor for the condition. Fatty liver isn't one of the central conditions necessary for the diagnosis of metabolic syndrome but it is almost universally present in people with the condition.

Now is an excellent time to tell you one of the principle tenants of this book: metabolic syndrome and fatty liver disease are both *reversible* because they are principally lifestyle related.

Fortunately, or unfortunately, depending on how you look at it, there is no pill available to treat either of these conditions. However, insulin resistance, metabolic syndrome and fatty liver can all be reversed to the point where they disappear. Read on to understand how.

Insulin is a hormone produced in the pancreas, which enables the body to use glucose as fuel. Insulin resistance means the cells in the body's organs don't respond normally to insulin's request to transport glucose from the blood into muscles and other tissues. Elevated production of insulin then ensues to try and resolve the impasse. Raised insulin levels from insulin resistance causes organ damage resulting in obesity, high blood pressure, high cholesterol, diabetes and metabolic syndrome.

These processes in turn then contribute to the development of heart disease, dementia, stroke, cancer, kidney failure and cirrhosis.

Throughout *Liver Better Life*, we'll come back to insulin resistance again and again.

The colonisers inside us

One of the leading theories explaining how some foods exert positive health effects and other foods create negative health effects is the interplay between the foods we eat and the bacteria in our gut. The scientific name for all of the bugs that live inside of the intestine is the gut microbiome.

The human gut is colonised by between 10 and 100 trillion microorganisms, mainly bacteria. In fact, the number of bacteria in our gut is greater than the number of cells making up our whole body. Although it's been known that the colon is populated with bacteria for centuries, it is only in the last decade or two that its role in health and disease has been explored by mainstream science.

In the womb, we don't have any bacteria in our gut. A baby's first exposure to microorganisms comes from their mother via the passage through the birth canal during delivery. Later the baby is exposed to more bacteria from breast milk and exposure to the environment. Gut bacterial populations, or gut flora, are often shared between family members. As our understanding of the potential role of gut flora in our health is evolving, it is emerging that this sharing of gut flora between family members may explain part of the shared health characteristics within families that has previously been attributed to genetics.

The gut flora in all of us is biologically active. It plays a role in food digestion and absorption, and generates many of the vitamins essential for health and vitality. These bacteria produce chemicals that protect the lining of the gut from injury and cancer. The flora is literally producing millions of chemicals, a biological soup that influences gut health and also health in general as many of these chemicals are absorbed across the lining of the gut into the circulation.

Gut bacteria and health

In a case of 'just in time' science, as we are recognising that exposure to bacteria in the environment is associated with good health there has been a proliferation of products promoted to sterilise the home environment, such as anti-bacterial sprays and hand washes. Added to this is 70 years of prolific antibiotic use, either to treat relatively mild self-limiting infections in people, or used in the livestock industry as growth promoters. Both household antibacterial products and direct antibiotic exposure result in a reduction of gut microbial diversity and potentially an increased risk of a variety of diseases.

Another interesting point to ponder on gut bacteria and health is pets. It is now well documented that pet owners are on average healthier than non-pet owners. Pet owners enjoy greater life expectancy, have fewer allergies and lower rates of mental illness. Historically this association has been explained by the benefits of companionship pets provide, as well as time spent exercising and outdoors with them. However, pet owners also have increased gut microbial diversity,[3] and the clinical benefits associated with pet ownership may relate to exposure to their bacteria more than the social benefits.

Bowel bugs, leaky gut and liver disease

It is well established that liver inflammation and fat are both common mechanisms for causing liver injury. Another mechanism of injury is leaky gut. Here's how it works. The gut is essentially a long hollow tube lined by cells. These cells are joined together by junctions that stop the contents of the gut spilling out into the surrounding tissues or directly into blood vessels. The gut is full of all sorts of health promoting chemicals, but also toxic chemical products generated from foods and bacteria. The gut cells are designed to cope with these products. But if they leak through the gut wall directly into the blood vessels then these toxic products travel directly to the liver where they cause liver fat accumulation and subsequent liver damage.[4] For a long time, it has been recognised that when the gut is sick, the liver gets damaged. Typically, this has been noted with gut-damaging diseases such as coeliac disease, Crohn's and colitis.

Over more recent years, research papers have suggested that the population of bugs that live in your gut, your gut microbiome, may also play a role in leaky gut. The proposed mechanism in this situation is that some populations of gut bugs are particularly prone to causing inflammation and damage to the gut wall. The gut bugs produce inflammatory chemicals that directly injure the gut wall, breaking down the tight cellular barrier that exists to protect the internal environment of the body from injury. These pro-inflammatory bacterial products then leak directly into the circulation and flow through blood vessels up to the liver causing liver damage.

Gut bacteria play a pivotal role in either maintaining liver health or causing liver disease. Recognising this is crucial because we are able to manipulate our gut bugs through what we eat. Probiotics will change your gut flora and metabolically facilitate liver health. I will talk about the data surrounding this issue later on. What you eat also has a significant impact on the populations of bugs in your gut. In general, a diet rich in a wide variety of fruits and vegetables allows the good bacteria in your gut to flourish and grow. A diet with high percentages of sugar and processed foods does the opposite. This feeds the 'bad bugs' in your gut and leads on to inflammation, leaky gut and liver damage. I will talk much more about what foods are good and which are bad in the subsequent chapters.

Earlier on I raised the premise that insulin resistance is one of the central driving forces causing liver injury and other consequences of the metabolic syndrome. Data is now emerging that ties gut flora and insulin resistance, some of the mechanistic pillars in our understanding of liver health/disease. An unhealthy diet can change the healthy population of bugs in your microbiome to an unhealthy one. The medical name for an unhealthy gut microbiome is intestinal dysbiosis. An unhealthy gut flora generates an inflammatory soup of chemicals in the gut. You may have heard discussions about a proinflammatory or anti-inflammatory diet. This effect of what we eat on our gut health is pivotal to our understanding of health maintenance and prevention of disease. This inflammatory environment damages the gut and is absorbed into the general circulation. This inflammatory cocktail from gut flora directly elevates insulin and contributes to insulin resistance. The use of probiotics in people with insulin resistance has been demonstrated to reduce insulin levels and improve insulin sensitivity.[5]

This is what's driving most diseases

Insulin resistance and intestinal dysbiosis (an unhealthy balance of bugs in your gut) are the pivotal mechanisms driving most of the diseases that affect Western populations. These processes in combination contribute to fatty liver, heart disease, stroke, diabetes and many cancers. There is a general misconception that, for example, heart disease has its own risk factors and cancer another list. Or that stroke and diabetes have totally different causes. The reality is that all of these diseases (and many more) share the same innate mechanisms.

This is conceptually important because the health information we receive can otherwise be very confusing. We are told, for example, to lose weight to reduce your risk of diabetes, to eat more vegetables to reduce your cancer risk and to exercise more to protect yourself from developing heart disease. These messages are all true but the reality of the overlapping messages is that it all becomes baffling. The simple truth is that all of these diseases are closely linked with the same driving pathological pathways. Preventing them or reversing them therefore also shares common interventions.

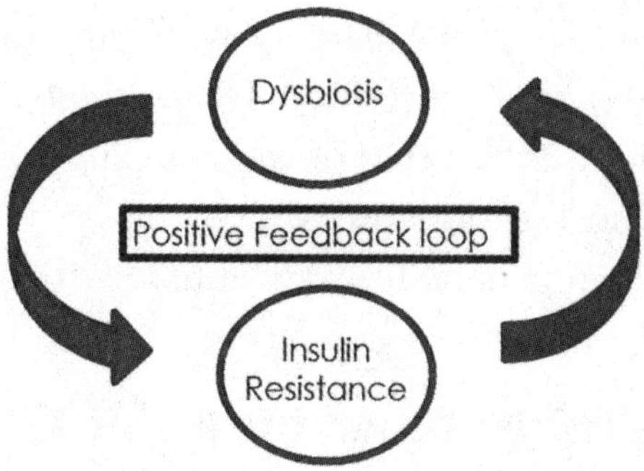

Figure 1.2 Insulin resistance and intestinal dysbiosis feed off each other, resulting in a positive feedback loop.

Insulin resistance and intestinal dysbiosis also feed off each other. Intestinal dysbiosis brews unhealthy chemicals in your gut which then get absorbed and result in inflammation in your blood. This then worsens insulin resistance. At the same time insulin resistance also directly changes your gut bugs, pushing them in the unhealthy direction towards dysbiosis. This creates a positive feedback loop which each abnormal process exacerbating the other. Fortunately both processes are reversible with the right lifestyle interventions. I will discuss these interventions in the following chapters.

GONER syndrome

As I have now discussed several times, the diseases that maim and kill most Western populations and many from the developing world share the basic drivers of insulin resistance and dysbiosis. You would expect therefore that there would be an umbrella term that described all these conditions. What is the term that ties in the diseases resulted from these shared mechanisms? Continually saying heart attack, dementia, stroke, diabetes, kidney failure and fatty liver disease becomes a mouthful after a while. Surprisingly there is no such term. So I'm going to make one to fill that void. GONER does this beautifully. It is very descriptive, isn't it?

GOw's syndrome of **N**asty **E**nergy dys**R**egulation.

Fatty liver is one of the best markers of your overall metabolic health. If you have fatty liver disease then you are on your way to developing one or more of the complications of GONER syndrome. Time to turn around now. If you get your liver health right, it is likely your general health will follow.

Thin on the outside, fat on the inside (TOFI) – could this be you?

Fatty liver is most often associated with being overweight, but as I mentioned earlier, we now know people who are ostensibly thin can still be carrying damaging levels of fat in their livers.

Fatty liver disease is extremely common and is almost always associated with a large waist and excess visceral fat. Yet nothing in medicine is ever absolute. You can have quite extreme levels of abdominal fat and still have a perfectly healthy liver. And you can have a small waist but still have fatty liver disease. It's typically abbreviated to TOFI: thin on the outside and fat on the inside.

The fat around your waist is made up of 2 discrete compartments: intra-abdominal fat (visceral fat), which is the liver toxic fat, and fat beneath the skin. Fat beneath the skin is called subcutaneous fat. In most people, the two are directly proportional. If you have a thin waist, you generally have small amounts of both visceral and subcutaneous fat. If you have a broad waist, you generally have excess visceral fat and excess subcutaneous fat.

Some people though, may have very little subcutaneous fat but still have excessive visceral fat and therefore still have fatty liver disease (TOFI). Fatty liver in people who are TOFI still causes liver injury and all of the other potential consequences of insulin resistance. And it is still completely reversible with the right lifestyle choices.

Everything else fatty liver can lead to

Cardiovascular disease, which includes heart attack, heart failure and stroke, is the most common cause of death in middle age. If you have fatty liver, your risk of developing cardiovascular disease is 350% that of the general population.[6] When you consider that cardiovascular disease is already quite common, those amplified risks should really be seen as unacceptable. But the bad news doesn't end there.

Fatty liver increases your risk of cancer. As we have discussed, an abnormally elevated insulin level is the primary mechanism leading to fatty liver disease. Insulin is also a growth factor. This may sound good, but it's not. Insulin stimulates the growth of fatty tissue and none of us want more of that. It also stimulates the growth of other tissues. In adults, this insulin-induced stimulus for growth can result in cancer. Liver cancer risk is markedly increased if you have fatty liver disease. Previously this association was thought to exist only for people who had liver scarring, but now we know that liver fat alone – the most benign end of the fatty liver disease spectrum – increases risk of liver cancer.[7] That's quite dramatic.

Cardiovascular disease includes heart attack, heart failure and stroke.
Ischemic heart disease refers to a heart attack.

The risk of developing other types of cancer also increases with fatty liver disease, especially bowel cancer. Already one of the most common cancers in our community, your risk of bowel cancer is multiplied by up to 5 if you have fatty liver compared to individuals who don't.[8] There is also preliminary evidence that fatty liver may increase the risk of cancers in the oesophagus, stomach, pancreas, kidney and breast.[9]

Yes, this data is distressing. But I'm determined you understand the reality – fatty liver has significant and serious consequences. And then there's diabetes; if you have fatty liver and don't already have diabetes, then you are at very high risk of developing it. Nearly one in 5 people develop diabetes within a few years of being diagnosed with fatty liver disease.[10] You may think obesity is the strongest risk factor for developing diabetes, but no, fatty liver is actually a better predictor of who will develop diabetes than overall weight.[10]

What doctors know and don't know

About now, you might be asking, if liver disease is so ubiquitous, and at the same time manageable, how have the medical profession let it come to this?

Some of the historical downplaying of fatty liver disease is likely due to paternalism; as the disease is extremely common, the medical fraternity don't want to create panic. It's difficult telling patients, 'You have a serious condition and I have no effective drug therapy to offer you.' It's only recently that there's been comprehensive data supporting the notion that lifestyle choices can literally turn this disease around.

Until the mid-1980s fatty liver wasn't even recognised. Nearly 40 years later many medical practitioners still don't understand it well enough. Doctors who completed medical school as recently as the 1990s were taught little or nothing about this condition during their medical degree. This gap in knowledge, understanding or focus wasn't intentional. Even with my specific focus on liver health, it's only in the last few years that I've really come to terms with what I intend to share with you via this book. So, let me explain why I think doctors have been slow to champion the changes you need to make to live long and well.

I was a medical student in the 1980s. We attended lectures on anatomy, physiology, biochemistry, behavioural sciences, pharmacology and many other topics. But there was no subject entitled nutrition. We studied how food is absorbed by the body and the diseases that can occur when there are problems with digestion or absorption. We had lectures on what makes up the basic components of foods – proteins, fats, carbohydrates, vitamins and minerals – but there was almost no analysis of the effects of diet on health and nothing on food quality. I expect this was true for most medical graduates, even those completing their degrees in more recent years.

After completing a medical degree, junior doctors spend many years in further training. To become a specialist physician in Australia it's at least 7 more years of ongoing clinical education. Junior doctors spend years at the coalface of patient care; in hospitals and general practices undertaking practical training on how to make a diagnosis from a patient's symptoms and signs. Junior medical staff spend years honing their skills at interpreting test results. They examine x-rays, CT scans, MRI, and all sorts of blood test data.

In addition, a lot of time is spent understanding and remembering the details of drug therapy for numerous conditions. It is clearly essential for doctors to be experts in prescribing and assessing drug therapy. Lots of time in training is devoted to acquiring this skill and experience. For many diseases, pharmacological therapy is the mainstay of treatment. If you have cancer or heart failure you want your doctor to be an expert in managing the drug therapy required for these disorders.

The majority of patients I see with a life-threatening condition are more than happy to take my advice about the appropriate drug therapy. After we have discussed the medications they need, most of them also ask about lifestyle measures that might help. For patients with non-life-threatening (in a shorter-term sense) conditions, lifestyle interventions are often the mainstay of treatment.

Here's the thing: despite the fact that most people who see a doctor for a serious condition request lifestyle advice, the majority of doctors are not trained or experienced enough on nutrition and lifestyle choices to provide patients with the information they need. This is no fault of the individual doctor – it is a result of how medical professionals are trained.

Why lifestyle factors get overlooked and are undervalued

So how is it that your doctor may have spent almost all of their training and focus on complex treatments, and not on learning more

approach to, fat in medicine and society. Let me be more specific: there are a number of risk factors for the development of fatty liver disease, which we will talk through in the subsequent chapters. However, the most potent risk factor is being overweight or obese. Historically, obesity was once an uncommon condition. As recently as the 1970s, less than 15% of children in Australia were overweight or obese; that rate now sits near 30%.[11] Since the 1990s, rates of obesity alone have increased by nearly 100%.[12] The inflexion point when rates of obesity appeared to lurch upwards worldwide happened in the mid 1970s.

What exactly caused this shift in the 70s is an active topic of debate in the scientific community. However, it is becoming apparent that the institution of dietary guidelines in the 1970s (that we are now recognising as flawed) are a significant contributor to the rising obesity rates since then. These dietary guidelines associated saturated fat with heart disease and suggested that saturated fat in the diet should be reduced and replaced with increased carbohydrates.[13] Fat was demonised and carbohydrates were the potential solution. Although the dietary guidelines also suggested increasing fruit and vegetables as the source of the additional carbohydrates this message was not clearly communicated or received.

Carbohydrate intake increased but primarily in the form of refined sugars. The dietary guidelines message coincided with a boom in the processed food industry. Carbohydrate-dense processed foods high in refined sugar slotted into the space left by 'bad fats'. Carbohydrates, especially refined carbohydrates, cause marked elevations in insulin levels. It is this hormonal consequence of the dietary change from fat to carbs that is one of the real drivers for the worldwide obesity epidemic of the last 40 years.

As this relationship becomes more broadly accepted, we will look back on this failed public health message of the 1970s as one of the greatest scientific health-related failures of the 20th century. Worldwide, it contributed to millions of deaths from heart disease, dementia, stroke, cirrhosis and cancers.

So that's the historic problem. However, even now, misinformation continues to cloud our responses to obesity and to individuals who need to manage their weight. For instance, many health professionals still understand obesity as a disease of kilojoule excess. This hypothesis is driven by the incorrect assessment that body weight is regulated by the balance between kilojoules in and kilojoules out. This system doesn't differentiate between kilojoules from ice-cream or kilojoules from lentils. A kilojoule is a kilojoule.

If this hypothesis were correct, kilojoule restricted dieting should result in weight loss. It is now absolutely clear to all who have tried and failed to lose weight and keep it off by dieting – and to anyone reading the scientific literature – that dieting does not result in significant long-term weight loss.[14] Loss of weight early in dieting is, of course, common. With time, however, the body becomes aware of the reduction in kilojoules and responds by reducing energy expenditure so as to maintain weight. If 'kilojoules intake' is reduced by 20% then the body will recognise this and compensate by reducing energy expenditure by a similar proportion. In this situation, a person dieting will feel cold (heat production is reduced), tired (energy levels are lower) and irritable. There may be an initial fall in body-weight but energy expenditure gradually falls to match this reduction in energy intake – and body weight gradually plateaus.

Hormones also undermine dieting efforts. During dieting the body's production of the hormones that control hunger rapidly and markedly increase. As diets continue, although body weight may have plateaued due to a fall in energy expenditure, hunger hormones are still much higher than baseline levels. Frequently, by 3 months into a diet, people start to gain some weight again due to their metabolic rate dropping to match energy intake and hunger hormones elevated compared to pre-diet levels. These mechanisms persist until body weight returns to pre-diet levels. In many individuals, weight gain may continue even after body weight returns to baseline. In the long term only a very small percentage of dieters lose weight and keep it off, and losses are generally less than 5% of baseline.[14]

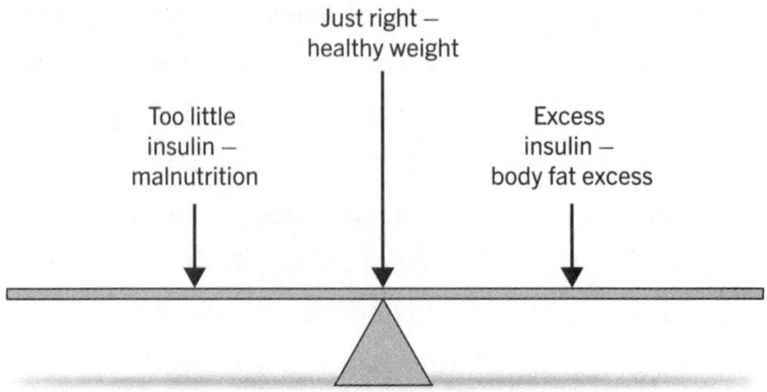

1.3a

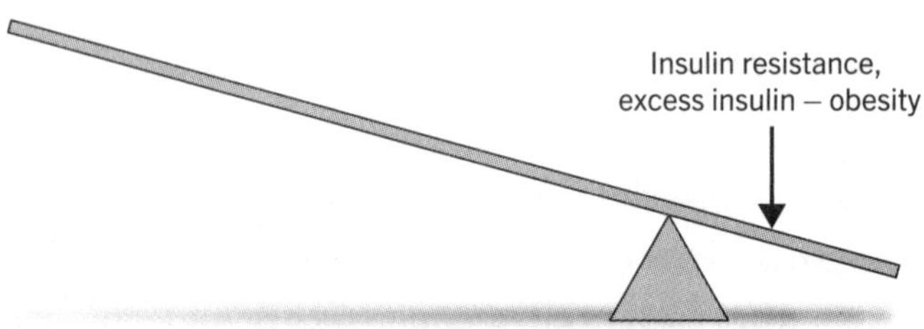

1.3b

Figure 1.3 Most people seesaw up and down a little bit from their own 'normal' weight (Figure 1.3a). However, long-term elevated levels of insulin reset the hypothalamus to higher and higher body weights, shifting the pivot point and creating a new normal in the individual often resulting in obesity (Figure 1.3b).

More recent is the hypothesis that obesity is a syndrome of insulin excess. As we know, insulin is the primary hormone involved in blood sugar regulation, and is released after eating carbohydrates. While insulin regulates blood sugar it also results in fat deposition. Chronically elevated insulin drives fat deposition and results in a gradual resetting of the body's weight fulcrum.

The part of the brain that regulates body weight in the long-term is the hypothalamus. Long-term elevated levels of insulin reset the hypothalamus to higher and higher body weight, creating a new normal for the individual. Dieting makes the hypothalamus reduce the metabolic rate so as to prevent weight loss. This is typically why diets don't work long-term. Many of the processed foods we all eat are advertised as low in fat, and that is true, but the fat is replaced with sugars, which are the metabolic culprit. Even low-kilojoule alternatives to sugar result in metabolic derangement, a phenomenon that will be discussed in depth in Chapter 4.

The long-term solution to obesity isn't about restricting kilojoules, but rather a long-term change in dietary composition to foods that result in lower insulin levels. Other important long-term interventions include rationalising meal timing, exercise, stress reduction and improving sleep quality. We'll talk about them all in the following chapters.

We don't have to go on like this

While the structural issues surrounding big pharma, money, research and education mean advances in our understanding of nutrition, health and disease are often overlooked, there is hope. Despite the fact that most major advances in medicine are driven by the pharmaceutical industry, there are still hundreds of new research papers published every day describing advances in our understanding of nutrition, lifestyle and health. While this progress doesn't receive the fanfare that drug-related advances do – and most medical professionals remain largely ignorant of the literature and science describing advances in our understanding of nutrition and health – we can change our own focus!

It's time to put history behind us and accept that fatty liver is a marker of premature death from a variety of other conditions. It is the warning sign, the canary in the coalmine that your body is under physiological stress. Rest assured, there's plenty you can do. The liver is a miraculous organ with tremendous regenerative capacity – fatty liver disease is completely reversible. By making the right lifestyle adjustments, your body's physiology changes; fat leaves the liver, any scarring that is there starts to repair and the risks associated with fatty liver disease resolve. The key is to listen to the message and react before too many of the potential complications have developed.

Chapter 2

Liver functions and dysfunction

The liver

For reasons I find hard to grasp, the liver doesn't have a reputation as the sexiest organ. The heart and the brain seem to get all the glory. But what is the heart, after all, but a simple pump; and the brain, isn't it just a computer? The liver however is astounding and wonderful. Like the heart and brain, the liver is a single, non-paired organ – so effective you only need one.

The liver resides in the right upper abdomen protected by the ribs. It is the largest of the body's solid organs – weighing about 1.5 kg in the average man and about 1.3 kg in women – and bright red, divided into 2 main segments or lobes; the larger right and the smaller left. The liver contains around 100,000 identical tiny factories called lobules. These lobules are the individual units that undertake all of the amazing chemistry that keeps you alive and well and your blood clean. Each lobule is made up of thousands of individual liver cells called hepatocytes. These cells have an average lifespan of about 6 months. The liver cells are continually dying and being replaced by new ones.

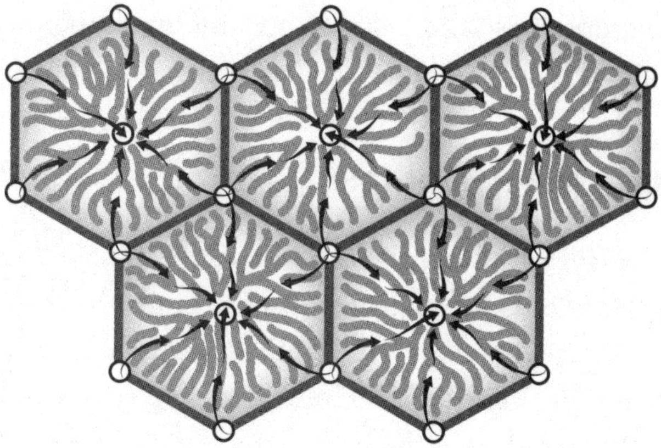

Figure 2.1 The liver is made up of one hundred thousand simple hexagonal units called lobules. The dirty blood from the gut enters the periphery of the lobule (hexagon) and flows along rows of liver cells where the blood is cleaned. The blood then exits the liver in the centre of the lobule (hexagon) and flows into the general circulation.

If you look at the liver under the microscope you can see the individual lobules are hexagons. Blood flows into the lobules from the outer angles of the hexagon and then centrally along rows of liver cells to a vein in the middle of the hexagon/lobule. This filtered and cleaned blood then leaves the liver and drains back into general circulation. The shape of the lobules is actually so dramatic and uniform that at first glance they don't appear to be natural forms. However, just as the hexagon of honeycomb fame (as well as snowflakes, the scutes of a turtle shell, the individual eyes of a fly or a raft of bubbles), these are hexagons brought to you by real life.

So why are the liver units hexagonal? The answer is stacked. When you stack spheres together, such as tennis balls, there is a large amount of space between the individual balls. In nature, this wasted space needs to be filled. There are only 3 shapes that can be stacked together with no space in between, the triangle, the square and the hexagon. Of these 3 shapes, the hexagon perimeter has the shortest total length compared with triangles or squares of the same area. So, bees employ the hexagon to save on the production of wax and

Mother Nature chose the hexagon for the liver lobules to save on space and energy in producing and replacing the individual units.

What does the liver do?

I think the real reason why the liver doesn't get all the love the heart and brain seem to is because most people don't understand what it does. We all conceptually understand what the heart and brain do. However, the liver's hundreds of individual functions can seem more nebulous. But put simply, the liver is the body's chemical factory; it gets rid of all the bad chemicals in our body and makes almost all of the good ones essential for life. Yet if the liver is a chemical factory, don't imagine it as a maze of steel pipes and chimneys spewing smoke and pollution. I see it more like a rainforest – making a wide range of exotic chemicals and cleaning the environment all at the same time. Or you could use the analogy of a native marshland, filtering the run-off from nearby mountains before the water splashes into a crystal-clear river. It's a beautiful thing.

Physically, the liver sits between your gut and the rest of your body. The positioning is important – in fact, perfect – as this facilitates the liver's filtering role between the gut and the body. The food we eat needs to be broken down into 'workable' units the body can use. This breakdown of food occurs in both the gut and the liver. Enzymes in our gut break down most of what we eat into tiny basic units so they can be absorbed. These are then transported across the gut wall into blood vessels. These blood vessels convey everything we've eaten directly up to the liver. This blood, and all the food products it carries, goes through the liver before it enters the rest of the body, so that hazardous chemicals can be removed and good chemicals retained and added. The liver also makes the body's blood clotting factors. These proteins are essential to make sure we don't bleed to death.

And the liver makes bile. Once produced, bile is sent down a tube called the bile duct to be stored in a reservoir – the gall

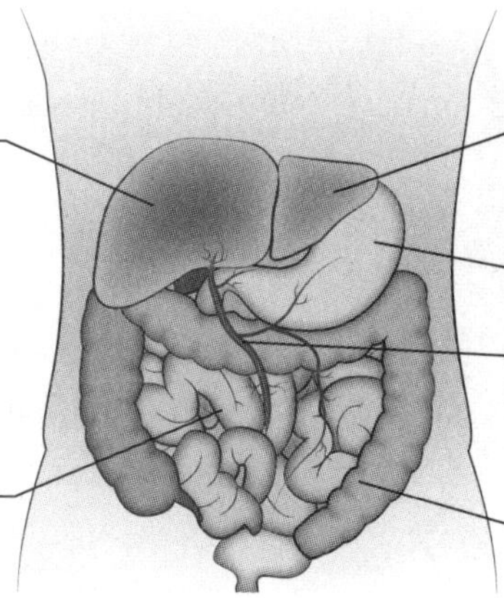

Figure 2.2 The liver lies between the gut and the remainder of the organs as a biological shield, protecting the body from gut derived toxins.

Just some of the liver's 500 functions

- Processing digested food from the intestine
- Controlling levels of fats, amino acids and glucose in the blood
- Clearing the blood of particles and infections, including bacteria
- Eliminating drugs and toxins
- Manufacturing bile to enable the body to absorb oily food
- Storing iron, vitamins and other essential chemicals
- Storing and releasing glycogen to produce quick energy
- Producing cholesterol
- Manufacturing the blood clotting factors
- Synthesising and regulating numerous hormones
- Making enzymes and proteins responsible for most chemical reactions in the body

bladder – until it is needed. When you have a fatty meal, the body detects the high fat levels and tells the gall bladder to contract. The contracting gall bladder squirts the stored bile out into the gut, to help with fat absorption.

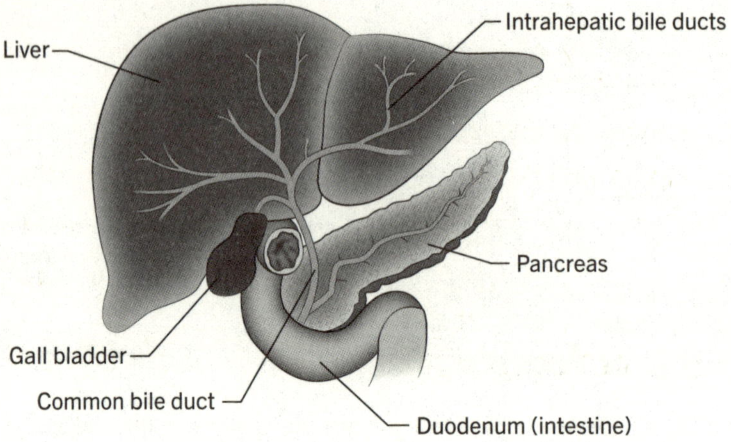

Figure 2.3 Bile produced in the liver flows down the bile duct into the start of the small intestine (the duodenum).

The liver also uses bile to eliminate waste chemicals. Once the liver has broken down all the toxic chemicals from the gut, it delivers these waste chemicals into the bile. The bile then goes back into the gut and the waste products are expelled from the body in the faeces. One major waste product that is excreted in bile is called bilirubin. Bilirubin is a yellowy/ brown colour and gives your faeces its colour. In some people with liver disease, the production of bile is reduced and one clinical consequence of this is that the stool becomes pale because the bilirubin pigment isn't getting from the liver into the stool. If you notice your stools are pale, it may be significant – get yourself along to see your doctor.

Some of the toxins normally excreted in bile (via the stool) can make you itchy if they aren't eliminated from your body effectively. So, if your liver is sick and not functioning effectively you may experience one of the classic symptoms of liver disease – itch. When the liver is sick or injured the excretion of these toxins into the bile is reduced and they accumulate in the blood. Liver-related itch typically doesn't create a skin rash, as the problem isn't in the skin, but the blood travelling through the skin.

Itch without a rash? It could be your liver!
Did you know?
In traditional Chinese medicine, the natural element aligned with the liver is wind, and itchiness is associated with 'wind' complaints.

The role of liver enzymes

The liver facilitates all of its smart chemistry via the production of substances called enzymes. Enzymes are chemicals produced by the body and are specifically designed to accelerate a chemical reaction. The liver makes hundreds of specific enzymes all designed to catalyse unique reactions. There are pathways of enzymes, for example, that turn simple sugars into glycogen. Glycogen is stored sugar that breaks down slowly overnight when you are asleep and/or fasting, which stops your brain dying from a lack of sugar. Enzymes also help make proteins for muscle, manufacture blood-clotting factors and facilitate excretion of nasty waste products such as ammonia.

In all of us – all the time – liver cells are dying and being replaced. When the liver is sick or fatty, the number of cells dying increases. When liver cells die they fall apart and minute amounts of liver enzymes are released into the blood. These can be measured. When your GP orders a blood test to gauge how your liver is working, these enzymes are measured and provide a general guide as to how healthy the liver is. This test is called a liver function test and is used to diagnose liver problems and measure the severity of liver disease.

The liver function test done by your GP actually measures the enzymes from dead liver cells in your blood.

Living with toxins

Every time we are exposed to toxins in food, they can potentially cause injury to the liver. Remember, most of what you eat is absorbed and then goes from the gut directly into the liver. The liver sits as a 'shield' between what you eat and the rest of your body. As we discussed previously, its location is no accident – it sits where it does to extract and utilise all the good stuff from the diet but also to remove all the toxins. The liver is highly efficient at removing toxins – but not perfect. As the blood from our gut goes through the liver, the liver is exposed to repeated minor bouts of injury from gut-derived toxins. Over the millennia of evolution, the liver has adapted to these repeated bouts of injury and simply recovers without any permanent damage. Indeed, the liver is renowned as the organ with the greatest potential for recovery and regeneration. It is this spectacular capacity for regeneration that allows the liver to recover even when it is severely damaged by fatty liver disease.

Medically, this potential for recovery after injury is utilised in a number of ways. If a patient has cancer in one part of the liver, this segment can be removed surgically. Instead of being left with a permanently impaired organ, the remaining liver will regrow over a period of weeks, returning to 100% of its pre-existing function. This capacity is also used in liver transplantation. In what's called living donor liver transplantation, it is possible to remove half the liver from a healthy person and transplant it into a patient dying from liver disease. In the donor, the liver will regrow to 100% of its normal capacity over weeks and in the recipient, similarly, the transplanted liver will regrow to a normal size. Essentially, making two livers out of one.

This capacity to recover is also why making changes in how you look after yourself, and your liver, is so powerful. If you give it a chance, your liver can regain its full level of function. After all, those liver cells replace themselves every 6 months. Every day is a chance to do right by your liver and leave it in a slightly better state. And as we've already seen, given all the jobs your liver performs, an effective liver will improve and support your longevity and life quality. So, there's plenty of good news! But before we go on to discuss what you can do to help your liver, let's take a look at what can happen when the liver is under stress for prolonged periods of time.

Liver disease – what goes wrong?

The liver is a remarkably resilient organ – it can take quite a battering before it gets really sick. However, even the almighty liver has its vulnerabilities. And strangely enough, while the list of things that can cause liver damage is quite long, most of them affect the liver in the same way. Things that are toxic to the liver cause inflammation in the liver and/or fat to be deposited. Inflammation, if allowed to persist for months or years, results in scar tissue accumulating in the liver. The scar tissue is deposited within the liver in a microscopic lattice-like fashion. If the amount of scar tissue reaches a critical level, a person is said to have cirrhosis. Fat deposited within liver cells can also result in inflammation and the same sequence of events – ending in scar tissue and cirrhosis.

Liver disease or liver damage initially appears as either inflammation or fat deposition.

When most people in Australia are asked what they think is the most common cause of liver disease, they generally answer alcohol. In fact, the most common cause is fatty liver disease. Some conservative authorities estimated that fatty liver disease affects more than 25% of Australians,[15] or more than 5.5 million people. Others put this figure at 50% of the population, although many of these cases are as yet undiagnosed. Fatty liver disease is one of the most common health problems in the Western world. The magnitude of this health problem worldwide is hard to comprehend.

Symptoms – could it be your liver?

In the majority of people, the first noticeable sign of liver disease is the development of excess visceral fat that typically occurs as people approach 40. As we discussed earlier, visceral fat (fat around the middle that encases the abdominal organs) is a potent cause of liver injury. Of course, it is very common for people to put on some weight as they approach middle age and none of us look on excess weight gain with any glee. However, where you put on the weight is vitally important. Weight gain around the waist is a very strong clinical marker that you have excess visceral fat and therefore may have fatty liver disease. Weight gain in other places such as the arms, legs and posterior may be annoying, but is less toxic to your metabolism.

An expanding waist generally means you have excess visceral fat. Visceral fat is the hallmark of insulin resistance, fatty liver and the subsequent complications of the metabolic syndrome.

It's important to take notice of weight gain on the waist, because for most people, there are no other easily discernible symptoms of liver disease until an enormous amount of damage and scarring has occurred. In fact, liver disease can take decades to cause scarring and cirrhosis, and patients may only develop other symptoms when they are a year or 2 away from death due to liver failure. The typical symptoms of liver disease occur very late in the course of the disease.

But just because you can't see it or feel it doesn't mean liver disease isn't deadly serious. When other symptoms do develop, the first to show up is most often excessive tiredness. But given that many of us – perhaps most of us – are tired, it's not an especially helpful flag. Tiredness in most people relates to being physically unfit, stressed, anxious, sleep deprived and probably to some degree is just part and parcel of the normal aging process. That said, symptom progression in liver disease typically starts out with feeling tired. This sense of exhaustion is the most common early clue of liver disease in both men and women. If tiredness is a new symptom for you, or if it is significantly impacting on your life, then take it seriously. So, if you need to have a regular nap, you can't get through your day without a lie-down or are struggling with your usual obligations at work or home, make an appointment with your local doctor and ask, 'Could it be my liver?'

Swollen ankles are another common early symptom of serious liver disease. As the liver gets sicker, the body retains extra fluid, and gravity means the fluid is most obvious around our ankles. But again, swelling around the ankles can occur with a variety of health problems, many of them quite benign, so just because your ankles are swollen doesn't mean you have liver disease, but it can be a clue. Another common symptom of liver disease is jaundice. Jaundice refers to yellow discoloration of the skin and the whites of the eyes.

The symptoms of liver disease tend to be non-specific and could be caused by other health issues making diagnosis complicated. Possible symptoms of liver disease include:

- excessive fatigue
- swollen ankles
- yellowing in the whites of the eyes
- yellow-tinged skin
- poor concentration
- holding fat around the waist
- itchy skin without an associated rash
- bruising easily.

One of the liver's basic functions is cleaning or filtering the blood, and liver damage makes it harder for the liver to perform this role. When the liver stops filtering the blood properly, toxins accumulate in the blood. Early on, while toxin levels are relatively low, people just feel tired or struggle to concentrate. Much later, toxins can accumulate to such an extent that they affect how the brain works. With these high toxin levels people become drowsy, then confused and ultimately unconscious.

The liver makes blood-clotting factors. These chemicals ensure your blood will clot effectively if you are knocked or bruised. If your liver is damaged, clotting factors are not produced in the necessary quantities and you will bruise very easily or get recurrent nosebleeds.

If you have any or all of these symptoms, then the first step is to speak with your local doctor and discuss your concerns that your symptoms may reflect liver disease. And then read on, because even as you follow the advice of your doctor, you can be instrumental in improving your liver health with simple adjustments to your diet and lifestyle.

How does your doctor assess your liver health?

If you've ever had a health check that includes blood tests, then almost certainly you have had a liver function test. A liver function test refers to a panel of blood tests to check the state of your liver. It is done if your doctor is concerned about your liver health, but more typically, as part of a general health assessment.

A liver function test typically checks 6 discrete chemicals. Two of these tests look at how your liver is working and measure albumin and bilirubin. The other 4 tests measure enzymes produced by the liver.

Albumin is a protein produced by the liver and is exactly the same chemical present in the white of an egg. When the liver starts to struggle, the production of albumin falls. One of the reasons this is important is that albumin's job is to keep the fluid within blood vessels in the circulation. When albumin levels are low, fluid leaks out of the blood vessels into the surrounding tissues. Gravity draws this fluid down and it collects around the ankles.

Bilirubin is a waste product – created by the liver from broken down red blood cells – which the liver excretes by squirting it down the bile duct into the bowel. Red blood cells have a finite life and are continually getting broken down. They contain a pigment (haemoglobin) that gives stool its characteristic yellow-brown colour. When your liver is struggling, the excretion of bilirubin is impaired and the bilirubin backs up in the blood and may be visible in the whites of your eye which take on a characteristic yellow hue. This is called jaundice. The body tries to eliminate the excess bilirubin in the urine, which takes on a tea or coke colour. Jaundice is concerning and can suggest quite serious underlying liver disease. However, nothing in medicine is absolutely black and white and bilirubin can increase for a number of other less concerning reasons.

The other 4 parameters measured in a liver function test are all liver enzymes. They are alkaline phosphatase (ALP), alanine aminotransferase (ALT), aspartate aminotransferase (AST) and gamma-glutamyl transferase (GGT). These enzymes aren't really measures of liver function (like albumin and bilirubin are). They are not measuring the efficiency of some special chemical reaction. In fact, they are all chemicals that are spilled into the blood when the liver is under stress. I view them as a measure of liver happiness.

Liver tests – the normal range versus the healthy range

With a healthy liver, all the chemicals measured in a liver function test should be in the normal range. However, what is defined as normal is set by the range of blood tests found in 95% of the healthy population. As we know, a quarter to half of the population have fatty liver disease (and this elevates these liver enzymes). Therefore, the accepted 'normal range' for liver function tests includes the results of 25–50% of the population who have fatty liver disease. So actually, a healthy fat-free liver should elicit test results which sit at the low end of the normal range.

One of the crucial and most important principles of this book is that these simple enzymes can predict your future. Liver function tests are markers of liver fat and insulin resistance. If your liver enzymes are way down in the low end of the normal range, then you have excellent liver health and it is likely that you will stay well in the decades ahead. If your liver enzymes are elevated, then almost certainly that is from liver fat. It may be that your liver is currently working fine – but it's a red flag that insulin resistance is developing, and your body chemistry is heading towards heart disease, stroke, diabetes and cancer. The time to intervene is when you are still well – rather than when the damage has been done.

ALT is one of the basic liver enzymes measured in a liver function test. For ALT, the healthy or normal range is anything below about 45 units/litre. The liver doesn't go from healthy to diseased in a stepwise fashion, there is a gradual transition. In this transitional area, or grey area, sit many people who have no obvious or definable liver disease and whose liver enzymes sit within the normal range, but at the upper range of normal. This really matters because even mild degrees of liver fat or inflammation are not benign – they are markers of insulin resistance.

Liver function tests are a marker of fatty liver and may be the best predictor of your future risk of developing many of the common diseases that lead to premature death in Western society.

Liver blood tests can predict early death

When you pool all the causes of premature death together, such as stroke, heart disease, cancer, cirrhosis and kidney failure, scientists term this all-cause mortality. As we have discussed earlier there is a shared pathology behind all these diseases: insulin resistance. Your liver enzymes are associated with your future all-cause mortality.

As you can see in Figure 2.4, the relationship between ALT (one of the basic liver function tests) and risk of death is 'J' shaped. The lower

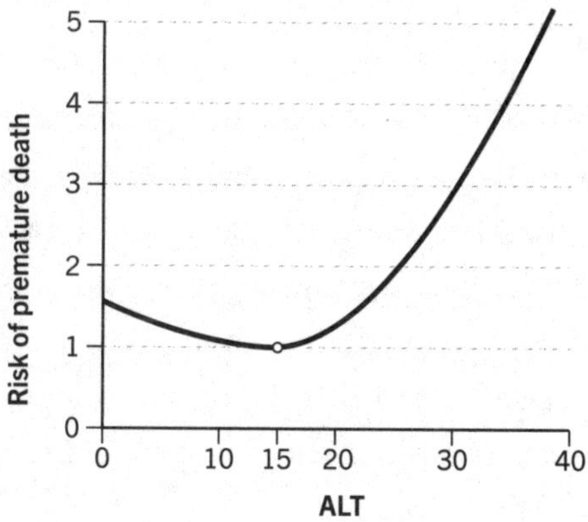

Figure 2.4 The relationship between ALT and risk of premature death.

limit of the J is an ALT of about 15. If your ALT is 30 (which is well within the normal range) your risk of death is about 2.5 times that of your peers with an ALT of 15. And if your ALT is 40, your risk of premature death is more than 5 times that of your peers with an ALT of 15.[16] That is quite a dramatic difference, especially given that all these results sit within the normal range. The explanation for this observed difference in rate of death is that ALT is a measure of metabolic 'wellness'. ALT measures minor degrees of liver fat and inflammation. This variation in liver fat and inflammation is a measure of your insulin resistance. If your liver fat is increased even a little you develop mild insulin resistance and your risk of liver disease, cardiovascular disease and cancer is elevated compared to someone with lower results.

Similar associations exist for the other liver enzymes. These liver enzyme measures are dynamic. If you address lifestyle issues, the numbers will fall, often dramatically.

Although there are 4 enzymes measured in a liver function test I don't feel one has greater importance compared with another when it is measuring metabolic distress from fatty liver. Physicians may spend years of their career exploring patterns in liver enzymes, but I feel for our purposes they are all really giving us the same message. If your results show high levels of these enzymes, it is less likely you will remain healthy as you get older. Do something about it.

Other liver tests

There are numerous other tests that can be ordered by your doctor to explore particular facets of liver health and disease, including ultrasound, CT scan, MRI scan, fibroscan and biopsy. These tests are used to explore specific questions a doctor has about the liver. If your liver function tests are elevated, then there are many diseases that might be responsible, and commonly your doctor will arrange further investigations to explore this for you. If the question is: Is there a liver cancer? Then ultrasound, CT scan or MRI may be used. If the question is: How much liver scarring is there? Then fibroscan, liver biopsy or MRI elastography may be requested. Fortunately for our purposes, the simple liver function tests are almost always adequate as a baseline measure of your liver health and metabolic wellness generally.

Below are some of my own ALT levels. Over the years they have trended up a bit but are all well within the normal range. My tests are pretty good – but there's still room to improve. From 2006 until 2013 I accumulated too much visceral fat from aging and inertia. With my improved lifestyle measures in recent years, my enzyme levels are falling and I'm on the way back to much better health.

Year	ALT level
2006	19
2012	21
2013	23
2019	20

Why isn't liver disease big news?

The last 3 or 4 decades have seen an explosion in medical science and research. Smallpox has gone. Polio is on the verge of eradication right around the globe. With many cancers, a cure is now not just possible, but expected. Rates of death from cardiovascular disease have fallen dramatically, but at the same time deaths from liver disease are increasing.

Diet and lifestyle issues play a central role in the development and treatment of almost all causes of liver disease. Despite the economic difficulties in performing non-pharma funded research, each year there are thousands of scientific papers published on aspects of diet and liver disease or liver health. However, the scientific community generally lacks either the skill or will to widely disseminate this information. Sadly, despite what may well be years of work by multiple researchers to generate one scientific paper, very often the novel information generated doesn't make it beyond the myopic world of one small area of science.

There's also the issue of how many health messages are delivered in brief bites in the media. With all the publicly available health information, it can be difficult to filter, balance and get the appropriate details and perspective. One day you hear that red wine is good for your heart, and the next day it isn't. How do you digest 2 apparently conflicting messages?

The lifestyle choices I am going to present in this book are the distillation of years of work from thousands of doctors and scientists who have contributed to the body of published works in this field. My aim is to present the sum of scientific evidence we have regarding diet, lifestyle and liver health. All the data presented here is extracted from published, peer reviewed sources and referenced scientific fact, not opinion. I have limited the data to published work relating to human health and have purposefully excluded work linking diet and liver health in other species as what may be true for rats may not be true for us.

For those of you who are reading more for curiosity – you've had the tests, and your doctor says you're in excellent health – you might be wondering if it's worth your time to focus on your liver. I say to you, if you already have a healthy liver, you can make it healthier, and feel the benefit for years to come. Read on.

Part 2

Liver healthy eating

Chapter 3

Can you eat your liver well?

Food. Is it just fuel?

Many people perceive food as simply fuel: basic vitamins, minerals and calories; energy for the engine. According to this logic, it makes no difference if those basic nutrients come from a jam donut or a bowl of nuts. Rationalised like this it doesn't matter what you eat, as long as you are getting adequate amounts of nutrients. Not too many and not too few.

However, what we need to recognise, as individuals and as a society, is that food is biologically active after we have eaten it. Food is not just calories or nutrients. Different types of food alter the way our whole body works, and change our insulin sensitivity. Although different foods such as donuts and nuts may well both have the same number of calories, the way your body reacts to these via insulin production may be vastly different. Remember from Chapter 1 – over-production of insulin is the enemy of your liver and your health in general. Sugary foods such as donuts will result in much higher levels of insulin in your blood than would a snack of nuts, even if the calorie content of both snacks were the same.

All foods impact insulin production to varying degrees. At its most basic, the magnitude of these changes determines whether you develop liver disease and other metabolic complications. The glycaemic index (GI) describes this phenomenon in the context of carbohydrate-containing foods. For the same number of calories, foods that cause a small rise in insulin levels are said to be low GI and foods that result in a large rise in insulin are referred to as high GI.

The figure below displays a useful model to keep in your head when making decisions about your health. When the pointer in the dial is turned to the left we are well; baseline insulin production is low, liver function is excellent and we are at low risk of all the 'aging' diseases. We can expect to remain well into our 70s and 80s. But when the pointer is angled to the far right the opposite is true. High levels of insulin and other growth factors causes obesity and increase your risk of liver damage, cirrhosis, cancer, heart disease, stroke, and diabetes (GONER syndrome). If your dial is pointed to the right you may anticipate being increasingly unwell as you age and either dying young or living your last decade or two infirm and frail.

Generally, the dial moves incredibly slowly. The way I think about it is, it takes thousands of decisions to move the dial from far right to the far left. What's important is the sum of many individual decisions that we make about our health. We all know it's nice to occasionally eat the wrong foods, be lazy, stay up too late and party into the wee hours. This is fun and can be good for us when it's an occasional

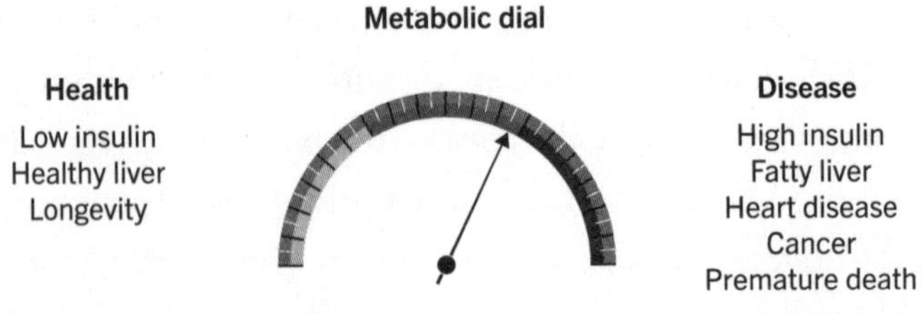

Figure 3.1 A concept of the metabolic dial that can oscillate between health and disease. The dial is very responsive to the lifestyle inputs of diet composition, weight, exercise, sleep and stress.

undertaking. It is the long-term, background, day-to-day decisions that determine where your metabolic dial is set and therefore how your liver health and general health will pan out in the years ahead.

The metabolic dial

Although I have primarily talked about insulin, that is not the only hormone exerting an effect on your body after you eat. Insulin is the best studied and most well known, but there are numerous other chemicals all exerting similar effects, including insulin-like growth factor-1 (IGF-1), growth hormone (GH) and hepatocyte growth factor (HGF). However, for the purposes of clarity and simplicity, I am going to keep the conversation primarily centred on insulin.

> One way food can influence hormones is by promoting growth. Growth may sound good – but is intrinsically bad! Growth directs the body to lay down fat in your tissues and liver. The primary hormone driving this is insulin.

Foods that result in large rises in insulin contribute to liver fat and scarring. The long-term consequences of eating these foods is that they drive our bodies towards growth (the bad kind), fat storage, heart disease, kidney disease, dementia and cancer. This metabolic impact of foods is largely independent of their caloric content. Some high-calorie meals will cause very small rises in insulin and drive our bodies toward health, while other foods relatively low in calories can have the opposite effect. This counter-intuitive message is integral to our understanding of a *liver better life*.

Foods that drive our metabolism in a healthy direction are the foods that form the mainstay of a liver-friendly diet. It may come as a surprise to many people that some of the foods and beverages that form the basis of this diet are foods we have traditionally associated as being 'bad' for us. Rest assured, looking after your liver doesn't mean a life resigned to kale and brussels sprouts.

Exactly what specific mechanism in foods allows some to exert beneficial effects and others a detrimental effect is extremely complex. And if we're talking *exactly*, we don't exactly know. Take coffee for example. We now know that coffee has significant positive health effects, specifically for liver health (so good for you in fact that I've devoted an entire chapter to coffee later in the book!). Coffee, however, is not just caffeine and water; it is made up of hundreds of different compounds, minerals, fats, sugars and proteins. So, is the health benefit related to one or two specific compounds in coffee? Or the ratios of some compounds to others, or just the sum total of the physiological effects of all the chemicals that exist in a cup of coffee? The answer is we don't know – and perhaps it doesn't matter as long as we know what is good and what is bad.

Poor dietary choices are now recognised to be the greatest risk factor for early death worldwide. The recently published Global Burden of Disease study looked at dietary composition in 195 countries over the last 3 decades.[17] The authors concluded that poor dietary choices accounted for one in 5 deaths worldwide, or 11 million deaths in the 2017 calendar year. Low intake of whole grains contributed to 3 million deaths annually and low fruit intake to 2 million deaths. The paper estimated that in Australia in 2017, 15% of all deaths were attributed to dietary risk. For all of us, a solid understanding of the health implications of our food choices is central to our future health.

Probiotics and liver health

In 2013, Vincent Wong and his colleagues from the Chinese University of Hong Kong published a simple but fascinating study that aimed to explore the role of gut bacteria in liver disease.[18] Vincent recruited just 20 people with fatty liver disease. Ten were given a probiotic every day (a capsule containing bacteria traditionally associated with gut health) and the other 10 recruits were given a placebo (dummy pill). The probiotic pill contained 2 different species of bugs with the predominant one being lactobacillus, the bacteria most commonly present in over-the-counter probiotics. Nothing else in the lives of the individuals was changed. Over the next 6 months he measured what happened to their liver blood tests and also the amount of fat in their livers. Liver function was measured using the simple blood tests I described in Chapter 2. Liver fat was measured using an MRI scan, which is a very accurate method. At the end of the 6-month period those who took the probiotics had reduced their liver fat by 30% and had markedly improved liver enzyme readings. Liver fat and liver function remained unchanged in those who took the placebo.

This study was not a one-off – there are now several similar trials demonstrating the same result. Probiotics somehow improve liver function and reduce liver fat. This sits nicely with our hypothesis that gut flora plays a major role in liver health. Probiotics contribute to liver health by promoting a biologically healthy soup of chemicals in the gut. This then aids gut integrity and minimises toxic chemicals leaking into the circulation and causing liver damage. Food does the same thing. Liver healthy foods feed good bugs, promoting gut integrity. Liver unhealthy foods feed 'bad bugs', resulting in leaky gut and liver damage.

It has also been reported that obesity, at least in part, relates to gut bacteria species and that obesity therefore may be transmissible[19] between individuals. The scientific literature contains a fascinating case that describes the apparent transmission of obesity in a woman who underwent a faecal transplantation.

In 2014 a 32-year-old woman from Rhode Island, USA, had recurrent diarrhoea for several months as a result of a Clostridium Difficile infection. When multiple courses of antibiotics failed, the woman was referred for a faecal transplant. While some people find the concept confronting, faecal transplantation is becoming standard therapy for patients with this specific gut infection that proves resistant to antibiotics. In Rhode Island, the patient's infection resolved soon after the transplant (that's the good news), but she gained 15 kg in the year after the procedure. As it turns out, the faecal donor was the patient's daughter who was in the middle of a period of rapid weight gain.

So, it seems your zoo of faecal microbes plays a role in your body's weight regulation and health generally. But how? Without doubt there are numerous overlapping mechanisms. Earlier I discussed how probiotics can lower insulin levels. What this implies is that 'bad faecal flora' increases insulin levels and promotes insulin resistance. Insulin then drives hunger and fat deposition.

Probiotics are live bacteria ingested for their beneficial effect on health.

Prebiotics are compounds in food that promote the growth of good bacteria in our gut. This is usually some form of fibre.

Synbiotics refer to supplements with a combination of probiotics and prebiotics.

One other mechanism whereby your faecal flora influences your body weight is by its effect on food digestion. Everyone's faecal flora is slightly different, just like a fingerprint. Within the spectrum of bowel bugs, some are better at breaking down food than others. In some people, fibre goes in one end and out the other. It is not broken down or absorbed and therefore you absorb no calories for it. In people with different gut bugs, this fibre is efficiently broken down by the bacteria. In the latter situation the energy released from the breakdown of the fibre is absorbed as additional calories resulting in weight gain, obesity, insulin resistance and fatty liver disease. In essence, some gut bacteria are better at harvesting energy from the diet than others.

It is becoming increasingly clear that our individual gut flora is an important parameter that plays a central role in controlling our body's metabolism. Having good gut bugs aids us in minimising weight gain and therefore helps protect us from fatty liver disease, diabetes, heart disease and cancer. Healthy gut flora is less 'inflammatory' and therefore will be protective against bacterial flora induced leaky gut and its contribution to liver disease. There are no doubt numerous factors that alter your gut flora, we have just talked about a few. These include your mother's gut flora, antibiotics use, household chemicals, gut infection, pets – and there will be many others. However, the most important factor that contributes to a healthy gut microbiome is your diet. Feed your gut bugs well and the good bugs flourish and in turn look after you well. Now we need to start looking at what is good, and what is not so good.

As you might be beginning to see, discussions that attempt to embrace gut flora, diet, general health and liver health show just how complicated the relationship between diet and health is. At this stage, it seems that diet influences gut flora, and diet and gut flora influence liver health. Conceptually this is important as it is a mistake to imagine there are foods that miraculously wash up through the liver and 'cleanse it' or others that do the opposite and damage it.

Food – what to eat and what not to eat for your liver

Does what I eat influence my risk of developing liver disease? Can I reduce my risk of developing cirrhosis by what I eat? Can I reduce my risk of developing liver cancer by changing my diet? These are all reasonable and important questions, and the answer to all of them is yes.

Now some more questions. Are there liver 'super foods' that will help my liver? What foods should I avoid if I have liver disease? Can different foods cleanse my liver?

It's taken me a while to get my head around the whole super-food concept. The medical tendency is to think of food in terms of protein, carbohydrates and fat, yet there's now plenty of science and large studies that show food is much more than those basic components. In the next chapters we'll discuss the benefits and potential risks of foods and diets in general, what you can do to protect your liver from disease if you have a healthy liver, and what you can do to help your liver if you have liver damage.

Are there particular foods that are bad for your liver?

The liver is an amazingly resilient organ and is primarily designed to break down all the chemicals we eat in our diet – and it does this extremely well. That means small amounts of almost all foods are handled without a problem by the liver. There is no one particular food that needs to be avoided in the pursuit of liver health. However, imbalances in the makeup of our diet can lead to or exacerbate liver disease. There are all sorts of urban myths that exist about diet in liver disease. Patients ask me frequently whether they should avoid meat. Should I be on a low-fat diet? Do I need to have blended fresh fruit juices? These are all myths! But there's plenty of science-based evidence that will allow you to improve your diet in support of liver health and longevity.

Chapter 4

Making room – ingredients to eat less often

Sugar

The average Australian consumes about 22 kg of sugar every year. A high-sugar diet has been linked to diabetes, obesity, heart disease, dementia and, of course, liver disease.

Sugar is the general term used for several different molecules of sweet carbohydrates found naturally in many foods. Processed sugar is used to artificially sweeten both processed foods and home cooking. It can be liver poison. There are, however, many different sugars, and some of these are good for us, and others metabolically toxic. I will spend quite a bit of time explaining how they fit into our diets, which are good and which are bad.

The 2 main types of sugar are referred to as simple sugars and complex sugars. There are 3 simple sugars which are individual molecules of sugar: fructose, glucose and galactose.

Commercially, the fructose added to processed foods is typically derived from sugar cane or corn. In nature, fructose may be found as an isolated molecule in fruit or it can be bound to a molecule of glucose to form the complex sugar, sucrose. Fructose is a naturally occurring sugar found in fruit, honey and most root vegetables.

Complex sugars are formed when 2 or more simple sugar molecules fuse together to form a larger molecule. These molecules can be 2 sugars fused together called disaccharides or multiple sugar molecules called polysaccharides.

There are 3 common disaccharides: sucrose, maltose and lactose. Sucrose is composed of one molecule of glucose and one molecule of fructose fused together. Sucrose is also the name for common table sugar. Maltose is 2 molecules of glucose joined and lactose is glucose and galactose joined together.

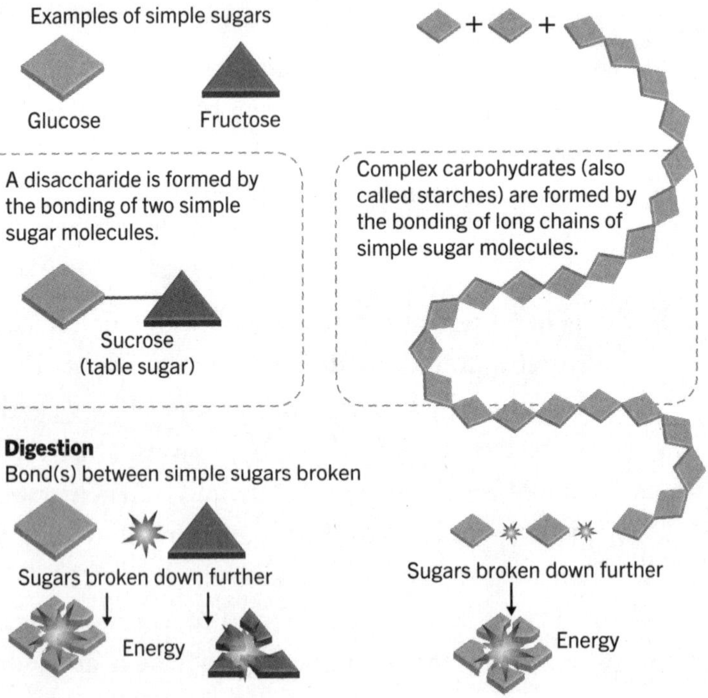

Figure 4.1 Types of simple and complex sugars.

Before being absorbed by the body, disaccharides and longer sugar molecules need to be broken down into individual sugars. We have enzymes in our small intestine that cleave the disaccharides sugar molecules into single sugars that can then be readily absorbed. Although there are numerous enzymes that may be involved in this process, we have evolved to produce specific enzymes to break down the disaccharide molecules into simple sugars for absorption. The enzyme that breaks down sucrose is called sucrase, the one that breaks down maltose is called maltase and the one that breaks down lactose is called lactase.

Galactose is a relatively rare simple sugar in natural foods. There are small amounts in some fruits, vegetables and nuts but most of the galactose in our diet comes from lactose (glucose and galactose) in dairy products. As it is a relatively rare sugar in our diet and is not used as an artificial sweetener I have no particular concerns regarding its role in liver problems.

The lactose issue

Sucrase and maltase are typically very efficient enzymes. They break down their associated complex sugars into simple sugars that can then be reliably absorbed. Lactase, however, is a different story. Lactose is the sugar in milk and other dairy products. Without enough of the enzyme lactase, lactose can't be properly broken down. As complex sugars such as lactose cannot be directly absorbed by the small intestine, the lactose passes directly from the small to the large intestine. The large intestine is designed to absorb salts and water from the stool. All the digestion of nutrients takes place in the small intestine. Therefore, when undigested lactose makes its way into the large intestine, the gut bugs that reside here make a meal of it. It doesn't do this quietly, however. The lactose is fermented by the gut bugs. Fermentation then results in the production of copious amounts of gas. This immediately leads to flatulence, bloating and gas-induced abdominal pain.

In addition, the sugars in the large intestine then act like an osmotic agent sucking water into the bowel causing diarrhoea. This sounds unattractive, I know, and it is. Lactose intolerance is not a disease but a variation of normal. It is common in many people all their lives and can also develop in individuals after gut infections, or just gradually with aging.

Interestingly lactose intolerance is very race-specific. Less than 10% of northern Europeans are lactose intolerant yet up to 95% of individuals in parts of Asia and Africa are. The hypothesis is that the ability to digest lactose offered a survival advantage to populations that domesticated dairy animals about 10,000 years ago. This domestication occurred predominantly in Northern Europe, but less commonly in Asia and Africa.

Lactose intolerance is not a condition associated with any harm. It can be a social inconvenience, but it is essentially benign. It definitely does not cause liver injury. Lactose is almost never added to foods and therefore is only a component of our diet when we eat dairy products. I will discuss dairy products and their potential health implications a little later in the book.

Fructose

Fructose has a number of adverse metabolic consequences that have implications for us all. The human body responds differently to fructose than it does to other sugars. For reasons that are so far unclear, fructose contributes to insulin resistance much more than other simple sugars.[20] Insulin resistance from fructose is not just due to the calorie load, but appears to be a specific metabolic effect of this sugar. With too much fructose, the body builds up high levels of insulin to combat the insulin resistance, and these higher levels of insulin results in visceral fat deposition around all the major organs, and fatty liver disease – and you know the consequences of this: GONER syndrome.

Fructose and body fat

There is a growing body of peer-reviewed scientific evidence suggesting that a diet high in fructose is strongly implicated in contributing to obesity, liver disease and its associated health problems. One such study followed 2 groups of individuals over a 10-week period. The first group was given drinks containing fructose as the sweetener, the other, drinks containing glucose as the sweetener. The aim was to see whether there was any difference in abdominal (visceral) fat accumulation over the 10 weeks between the 2 groups. Although the sugar type was different between the 2 groups, the calories in the drinks were the same. This design allowed the investigators to ensure any difference in fat accumulation at the end of the study couldn't be attributed to differences in caloric load.

The scientists found that the group who drank the fructose-containing-drinks gained more abdominal fat[21] – in fact, more than 4 times the fat gained by the individuals drinking glucose sweetened drinks! In addition, the fructose group gained more liver fat and became more resistant to the effects of insulin.

Some in the industry continue to argue that fructose only contributes to problems when people consume too much. They claim that if people stayed within their ideal calorie guidelines then fructose won't cause a problem. It's an interesting hypothesis. One lovely thing about science is that if you can clearly define a hypothesis, then you can design an experiment to explore it. Richard Johnston from the University of Nottingham is one such clear-thinking scientist. He designed an experiment where 32 chubby but healthy men had a diet either high in fructose or a diet high in glucose, but with the overall calories in their diets still falling within the healthy range.[22] This experiment explored whether a diet high in sugar (either fructose or glucose) but with a healthy total calorie count contributed to liver fat and insulin resistance. Richard found that the high-fructose diet markedly increased insulin resistance whereas the diet high in glucose did almost nothing. In this study, liver fat remained the same. So even if you don't eat too much, a diet high in fructose contributes to metabolic dysfunction much more than a diet high in glucose.

Richard explored a second hypothesis within that same study. He gave the participants a break from the study for 6 weeks then invited them back for a second dietary intervention. This time he again gave the men a diet high in either fructose or glucose, but he also asked them to eat as much as they could. The aim was to explore the effect of the 2 sugars when they are part of a diet containing excessive calories. Richard found that weight gain and liver fat increased in the men given both fructose and glucose. What this means is that if the total calories in your diet are in the healthy range then fructose is bad for you but not necessarily glucose. However, if you eat too much, then both fructose and glucose are equally bad.

So, fructose appears to preferentially contribute to abdominal fat accumulation and insulin resistance – and insulin resistance is the start of the cascade that leads to liver fat, heart disease, cancer, and the end.

In a Danish study,[23] participants who were overweight but had healthy livers were allocated a particular drink for 6 months. The aim was to compare the impact of certain beverages on whether people developed fatty liver disease during the 6 months of the study. People were assigned to either Coca-Cola (high sucrose and therefore high fructose), milk (which contains lactose and had the same calorie content as the Coca-Cola) or Diet Coke (no calories). What they found at the end of the study was dramatic. Those who had the milk didn't develop fatty liver disease. Neither did those who drank Diet Coke – nothing happened to the liver. However, for those who had the high-fructose Coca-Cola diet, liver fat increased by 140%. This is really a wow moment when examining the connection between what we put in our mouths and liver disease. It's not just too many calories that causes liver disease – but the form of the calories.

A similarly powerful piece of data comes from a relatively small North American study of adolescent boys. Forty boys between the ages of 11 and 16 who all had fatty liver were included in the study. Half continued their normal diet (the control group) and the other half were supplied with a diet that had the same number of calories as the control group but less than 5% of the calories came from sugar. It isn't specified in the study what the sugar was, but it is implied that it is sucrose (a mix of fructose and glucose). Five percent of the calories in the diet coming from sugar is a very low intake.

After just 8 weeks of this change there were dramatic improvements in liver fat in those undertaking the low sugar diet. Liver enzymes improved significantly, and liver fat fell markedly. The results of this study help stitch up the central role sugar plays in contributing to liver fat. It is not calories that are necessarily to blame – it is the form the calories come in. Sugar is bad. Also, the study illustrates how quickly things can turn around. In just the 8 weeks that these individuals changed their diet, liver fat fell by 30%.[24]

So metabolically, fructose seems to typically make people fatter than other sugars. Also, fat gain associated with fructose sweetened foods doesn't just go on anywhere; it is typically visceral fat, the dangerous fat. Fructose doesn't just contribute to the accumulation of visceral fat and liver fat, it also looks like our brains may respond to fructose differently than other sugars, making it harder to feel satisfied after eating. Lower levels of satiety (the feeling of fullness), mean we eat more, even excessively.

A team of researchers led by Professor Christoph Beglinger from Basel, Switzerland set out to explore whether fructose affected the brain and its signals of satiety differently to glucose.[25] The researchers enrolled 12 healthy young men who had nasogastric tubes inserted and a 250 ml infusion instilled into the stomach of either fructose, glucose or a placebo. The researchers asked the participants to score their feeling of satiety, measured their satiety-hormone levels and did functional brain MRI scans. The results revealed fructose and glucose affect the brain quite differently.

Satiety-hormone levels in the blood were lower for the fructose group, and participants reported feeling hungrier as well. What this data implies is that fructose-containing foods are less good at telling you to stop eating.

The great majority of people with fatty liver disease are overweight, generally with excess visceral fat. So can a high-fructose diet cause fatty liver if you are lean? One of the leaders in this field thinks so. Dr Nimer Assy from Ziv Medical Centre, Israel is an expert on dietary composition and fatty liver disease. To explore the potential causes of liver damage in lean people with fatty liver, Dr Assy and colleagues collected detailed lifestyle and dietary information every 6 months over a period of 3 years from a group of 31 such individuals.

Dr Assy's findings suggested the likely cause of liver damage in this group was a diet high in fructose-containing soft drink. Eighty percent of the lean people with liver disease consumed an excessive quantity of soft drink. On average, this group consumed more than 450 ml of soft drink daily, which means 50 g of sugar. Importantly, the association between liver damage and fructose-containing drinks was independent of exercise and other potential lifestyle factors.[26]

If I have fatty liver disease, does fructose make it worse?

You guessed right – yes. The medical evidence suggests that if you have fatty liver, a diet high in fructose increases the chance of progression to severe scarring and permanent liver injury.[27]

The potential impact of a high-fructose diet on other liver diseases is still being assessed by the scientific community. However a study on people living with hepatitis C reported they had much more severe and permanent liver injury if they had a diet high in added non-fruit fructose, whereas the naturally occurring fructose in fruit made no difference to people's liver disease.[28]

Fructose is in fruit – how can it be bad for you?

To be reassured that a diet high in fructose from fruit is safe from the metabolic damage seen when foods are artificially sweetened, scientists gave well people a diet very high in fruit and measured what happened to liver fat. The results came as no surprise. Fruit is good. The study in question was performed in Sweden and published in 2016.[29] The design was quite simple: 30 well people were recruited and had their normal diets supplemented with either a large amount of fruit (the equivalent of about 7 apples per day) or a diet with extra nuts of equal calories (70 g of walnuts). As the aim of the study was to explore whether added fructose from fruit is bad, the control group got added calories from nuts (no extra fructose). At the conclusion of the 2-month study period liver fat and visceral fat was measured by MRI in both groups. The conclusion of the study was that liver fat and visceral fat were unchanged in both groups. A diet high in fructose from fruit does nothing bad to you, your metabolic profile or your liver fat. It is clear that fructose from fruit is fine, fructose added to sweeten foods is bad.

Fruit is a wholefood

We also know that fructose in fruit appears to act differently than fructose/sucrose added as a sweetener to foods. Fruit is more than just fructose, vitamin C and water. Fruit is full of large quantities of chemicals called polyphenols. Polyphenols are plant-based chemicals that exert important positive metabolic effects, and in many ways have the opposite metabolic outcome of fructose. Polyphenols reduce insulin levels, make the body more sensitive to insulin, reduce liver fat and reduce intra-abdominal fat. The fact is, fructose delivered in an apple or an orange is not at all comparable with fructose in soft drink.

Here's the 'to do list' when it comes to avoiding fructose

- Avoid fast food – sucrose and fructose are often added to fast food as a sweetener
- Avoid soft drinks – they are high in fructose and offer no nutritional benefits
- Avoid artificially sweetened fruit juice (usually sweetened with sucrose, which contains fructose)
- Buy fresh foods and learn to cook
- Remember, sugar is poison, and foods with added sugar are not your friend
- Start reading food labels – it's empowering
- Spend more time shopping around the edge of the supermarket than the middle – fruit, vegetables, grains and dairy are around the edges, whereas processed foods (typically artificially sweetened) in packets and jars are in the middle

How much sugar is too much?

When it comes to refined sugar, not sugars in fruits and dairy, how much is too much? Well, this depends on who you talk to. And when.

According to the World Health Organization (WHO) less than 10% of our total calories should come in the form of what they call 'free sugars'. Free sugars are simple sugars that have been added to foods, not sugars that occur naturally in fruit and vegetables. This equates to about 50 g of sugar daily – or about 10 teaspoons.

WHO also suggests, that ultimately, we should be aiming for 5% or less of our calories to be free sugars (25 g daily or 5 teaspoons). Five teaspoons may sound like a lot, but it is very easy to consume this because sugar is added to almost every processed food or drink you buy. A can of Coke or Pepsi (330 ml) contains about 35 g of sugar – there's 8 teaspoons right there!! – and most popular soft drinks have just as much or more.

Fruit juice, bread, breakfast cereal, fruit bars, sauces and biscuits are all commonly high in sugar. Although it is a safe assumption that all processed foods are likely to contain some free sugars, it is surprisingly hard to predict which are going to contain large amounts. This is where you need to read the label. Avoid foods where the sugar content is high. Although it is hard to define what high is, when the percentage is greater than 10% I start to look for lower sugar alternatives.

The WHO guidelines do not differentiate fructose from other simple sugars. It seems likely that with small amounts of free sugars (less than 5% of calorie intake as advised by the WHO), there is little difference between fructose and other sugars. However, with larger amounts of free sugar (>10%), fructose is associated with greater liver damage and metabolic consequences than other sugars.

Artificial sweeteners

I was a fan of Coca-Cola for many years. I enjoyed a can with lunch most days of the week. Over the hotter summer months, I drank even more. It was a reward after toiling in the garden for hours or after returning from the beach. But about 15 years ago I realised, after decades of being skinny, that I wasn't thin any more. My waist circumference grew and my belt needed to be let out a notch. I was developing a belly. Just a little belly, but it was there. My mother-in-law is Spanish and she described it as a barriga. That's the endearing Spanish word for chubby tummy. Barriga is a much nicer term than beer belly. The South Africans call it a boep, also a great word.

But cute words didn't make it okay, so to get rid of my barriga, I decided to ditch Coke and move to Diet Coke. This was difficult – as I am sure some of you know – but it made me feel virtuous. I could drink it without liver recrimination. I assumed this would tame my barriga in years to come, since Diet Coke has no calories.

So I continued my relationship with Diet Coke up until the last few years. And while I recognised it as a vice, of sorts, I believed there was no associated liability. But I am now in the process of severing the thirst forever, although it's been a slow process. I felt it was necessary to break this habit because the emerging scientific message says that artificial sweeteners are not metabolically inert. In fact, the latest evidence suggests that instead of being a solution for obesity and its associated complications, artificial sweeteners may in fact be contributing to the problem.

The body's normal response to a sugar-laden drink or meal is to release hormones that reduce appetite. This of course makes sense; your body is satisfied with the sugar hit and doesn't need any further calories, at least for a number of hours. At face value, it may be reasonable to expect the same response with a drink containing artificial sweetener. But that's not the case. After a drink containing these chemicals, there is no hormonal response from the body to switch off appetite. Although your taste buds recognise a sweet drink, your body knows it's getting a calorie-deficient substitute – and appetite is not satisfied. There is even some evidence to suggest that the ingestion of artificial sweeteners is associated with a heightened hunger response. This implies that at the next meal, your body will be asking for more than it otherwise would have.[30]

Artificial sweeteners are also associated with an increased risk of fatty liver, diabetes and obesity. Here it can be difficult to know what is cause and what is effect. Do people concerned about a deterioration in their health change to diet drinks or do diet drinks themselves contribute to the health problem? To help resolve this very important question, Jotham Suez and colleagues from the Weizmann Institute of Science in Israel explored the issue.[31] Their study was published in *Nature*, a prestigious and highly respected scientific journal. To explore the hypothesis that artificial sweeteners are associated with the development of insulin resistance, the authors designed a relatively simple experiment. Seven healthy young people who didn't normally consume artificially sweetened drinks were given high doses of saccharine (an artificial sweetener) for 6 days. The researchers then measured blood sugar as a short-term measure of insulin resistance/metabolic syndrome. What they found was profoundly concerning. Four of the 7 individuals developed insulin resistance/metabolic syndrome within days of exposure.

Although the above experiment by itself has very important implications, Dr Suez and colleagues went on to perform a second experiment on the participants. Stool samples were analysed from the 7 participants with the researchers hypothesising that the mechanism by which artificial sweeteners induce metabolic derangement was via the development of abnormal gut flora. Indeed, after exposure to artificial sweetener for just a week, changes to the gut flora had occurred in the 4 people who developed metabolic syndrome markers. Little change was seen in the other 3 – suggesting there is some individual variation in response to these products.

Not satisfied that their job was complete, Dr Suez and colleagues designed one further experiment. They wanted to know whether the changes in participants' gut flora was the cause of metabolic syndrome. To resolve this question, the gut flora from the participants was transplanted into mice that were bred to have no gut flora, called germ-free mice. What was found was that when germ-free mice received gut flora from people with artificial-sweetener-induced metabolic syndrome the mice developed metabolic syndrome. When germ-free mice received gut flora from participants who didn't develop metabolic syndrome, the mice didn't develop metabolic syndrome.

This data concerning artificial sweeteners is rich and important and worth distilling. The first point to emphasise from the experiments we have discussed is that these chemicals have metabolic consequences. Artificial sweeteners may not have calories, but they cause changes to your metabolism that are similar to the changes seen with a high-fructose diet. This may seem surprising that calorie-free food can cause changes to your metabolism similar to a high sugar diet. But this is the point. What happens to your liver health, metabolism and weight is not as simple as calories in and calories out. Different foods affect your liver health and metabolism markedly differently. A 1,000 calorie meal of vegetables is likely to contribute to liver health and protect you from metabolic syndrome and obesity. A 1,000 calorie meal of sweet donuts will do the opposite. And a zero calorie diet drink may have similar adverse health effects.

The metabolic effects of food are partly independent of its calorie content. Foods exert their impact on your metabolism partly via changing your gut flora. This was demonstrated nicely in the artificial sweetener study we discussed earlier. Gut flora can help create a healthy liver, lean waist and offer protection from metabolic syndrome. Or a change in your gut flora can be bad for you. As discussed in Chapter 1, the medical term for bad gut flora is dysbiosis. Dysbiosis can result in gut inflammation, leaky gut, liver damage, visceral fat deposition and metabolic syndrome.

Chapter 5

Food, glorious food!

The Mediterranean diet

Several millennia ago, the area surrounding the Mediterranean was populated by the Greeks, Romans and the Phoenicians, who shared farming and culinary skills based around wheat, olives and grapes. Over time, these foods evolved to become bread, wine and olive oil. These 3 central components make up the backbone of the modern Mediterranean diet. Fruit and vegetables form the other cornerstones of the diet and, even today, anyone visiting traditional markets from Morocco to Palermo will have their senses overwhelmed with the cornucopia of fresh tomatoes, garlic, figs, artichokes, wild greens such as dandelion leaves, herbs, cucumbers, eggplant, beetroot, fennel, celery, lemons, lettuce, mushrooms, nettles and zucchinis.

The Mediterranean diet is the modern name given to the traditional diet of the southern European countries of Italy, Spain and Greece. Although, with more than 20 countries surrounding the Mediterranean Sea, there is marked variation in eating habits and dietary traditions. The Mediterranean diet and its association with health was first recognised more than 40 years ago.[32] The Seven Countries Study in the 1970s was the first large-scale research project to explore the hypothesis that lifestyle and diet were risk factors for heart disease. It seems amazing in the 21st century, when we innately accept the link between diet and cardiovascular health, to think there was a time, not that far back, where this seemed a radical hypothesis.

The study enrolled people from the USA, Japan, Finland, Yugoslavia, Netherlands, Italy and Greece. Parts of the study continue even today. What quickly became obvious was that deaths from heart disease were much more common in the USA and Northern Europe compared with Southern Europe – even after adjusting for age, cholesterol, blood pressure, smoking, weight and physical activity. One of the study's conclusions was that the diet of Southern Europe appeared to protect against the development of cardiovascular disease.

The Mediterranean diet typically consists of a *lot* of olive oil, legumes (beans), fruit and vegetables; moderate servings of fish, dairy products (mostly as cheese and yoghurt) and alcohol; and small amounts of meat. This approach to eating is relatively high in fat – but associated with a low risk of cardiovascular disease. But in truth, the high fat content of the Mediterranean diet is perhaps one of its greatest joys. Not because it's naughty, but because it brings a salad to life encouraging eaters to savour food, and supports health in a multitude of ways we are yet to fully understand.

Via the Seven Countries Study, the researchers compiled compelling evidence that the Mediterranean diet protects against heart disease; however the benefits aren't limited to the heart. Eating this way improves liver health, reduces the risk of diabetes, lowers blood sugar levels, and reduces levels of cholesterol and triglycerides while increasing good cholesterol.[33] It protects liver health and defends against the development of the metabolic syndrome. It also reduces inflammation and the risk of blood clotting and increases antioxidant activity. Both the science and logic point to the Mediterranean diet as the dietary trust for liver health.

The evidence for the Mediterranean diet in liver disease

In the medical scientific literature, the gold standard for proving something works is the randomised controlled trial. A randomised controlled trial is where you have 2 groups of patients with a disease. Half get the new intervention (a pill – or in this case a diet) and the other get a placebo (dummy pill, or in this case their standard diet); and at the end of the study the results of the 2 groups are compared. There are now several small, randomised controlled studies that explore different effects of the Mediterranean diet on liver health, with all being positive.

The seminal study exploring the effect of the Mediterranean diet on liver disease was undertaken by Dr Marno Ryan from St Vincent's Hospital in Melbourne. The study recruited just 12 people for a 6-week study – all had fatty liver disease. Six of the 12 were put on the Mediterranean diet and the other 6 followed a standard low-fat diet. At the conclusion of the study, MRI scanning revealed that those on the Mediterranean diet had reduced the fat in their liver by an average of nearly 40% compared to their baseline – those on the standard diet had reduced liver fat by just 7%. Importantly, the group on the Mediterranean diet had not lost any weight. This could be perceived as a negative for the study – but it is actually scientifically very important. The fact that liver fat improved markedly while weight stayed the same suggests the reduction in liver fat was not due to weight loss but due to a change in the body's metabolism that was independent from weight. The diet changed the way the whole body worked for the better. Yes, this is just one study and, yes, it's small but it does fit with the weight of evidence that suggests the Mediterranean diet is especially good for liver health.

In a Melbourne-based trial, adherence to the Mediterranean diet delivered a 40% reduction in liver fat in 6 weeks – without a loss in overall body weight.

I have previously made the point that weight gain and calories are not directly related. Of course, they are connected, but it is not a one-to-one assocation. The type of food you eat is crucially important in your body's response to it. Some foods are much more likely to cause weight gain than others. The results from Dr Ryan's study add further to this theme. What she has shown is that dietary composition, not just calories, influences your liver health and measures of the metabolic syndrome. This principle makes it crucially important for how you look at food for the rest of your life.

Mediterranean diet and fatty liver disease

One of the issues with randomised controlled trials and medicine is that the timeframe is often very short – in Dr Ryan's study it was just 6 weeks. This isn't long, given liver disease often progresses over years or decades. What is important therefore, is data that examines whether the Mediterranean diet can reduce the risk of developing cirrhosis or liver cancer, which are the long-term end-points of liver disease. Dr Ryan's trial showed that following the Mediterranean diet reduces liver fat; but what we really want to know is whether the Mediterranean diet is going to reduce the risk of dying from liver disease.

Well, actually, we do have long-term data that addresses this question. How individuals apply the dietary principles of the Mediterranean diet varies markedly. However, the scientific evidence is that the closer your diet is to the ideal Mediterranean diet, then the lower your risk of liver cancer – and this relationship appears to be linear. What this means is that people with an ideal Mediterranean diet have a risk of liver cancer half that of those on a non-Mediterranean diet – and those with a moderate Mediterranean diet having a risk somewhere between the two.[34]

Even more compelling, emerging evidence suggests that a non-Mediterranean diet also appears to increase your risk of dying from liver disease. Wen-Qing Li from the National Cancer Institute, Rhode Island, USA has examined just this hypothesis.[35] Wen-Qing Li explored a database of dietary information of nearly half a million North Americans. His data revealed that the further away from a typical Mediterranean diet you are, the more likely you are to die from liver disease or liver cancer.

I'm saying it loud: the Mediterranean diet reduces markers of inflammation, has beneficial effects on blood cholesterol, reduces your waist circumference and reduces the risk of diabetes. Inflammation and insulin resistance are the basic drivers of fatty liver disease; the beneficial effects of the Mediterranean diet reverse these pathological processes.

One of the premises of this book is that to lead a *liver better life* you don't need to be a monk; you don't need to miss out on the dietary pleasures of life. Indeed, if you are living a life of gastronomic abstinence you are probably doing your liver more harm than good. As we will discuss later, coffee and alcohol (in moderation) are some of life's simple pleasures and are good for your liver – and for your health generally. On the same theme, the Mediterranean diet, although relatively high in fat, is pleasurable to eat and offers significant benefits for liver health and overall health. This may seem counter-intuitive, but there it is; it's good for you.

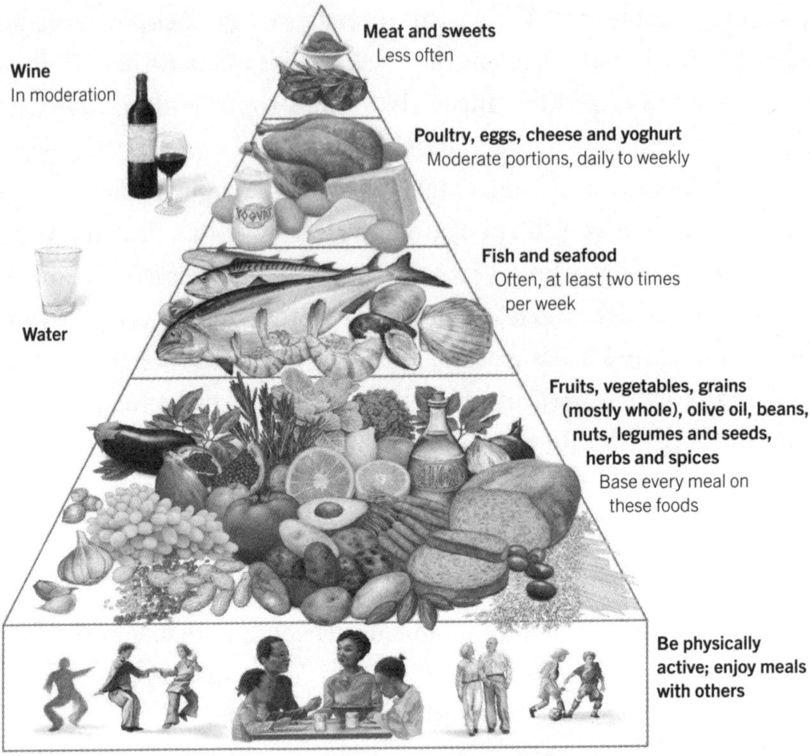

Figure 5.1 The Mediterranean diet. Feel free to eat lots of what is at the base and less of the foods at the apex of the pyramid.
© 2009 Oldways Preservation & Exchange Trust, www.oldwayspt.org

The Mediterranean diet in depth

The original authors of the Seven Countries Study noted that the farmers of Crete consumed a diet very high in fat, yet had the lowest death rate from heart disease. Heart disease is relevant to us because it is a marker of metabolic syndrome. Even in 2021, this seems counter-intuitive. We have been sold the message for over 40 years that fat is bad for us, and we have avoided it. And while avoiding fat we have increased our intake of sugars – most notably fructose artificially added to foods. This has contributed to the rise in fatty liver disease, insulin resistance and all the manifestations of metabolic syndrome. We need the Mediterranean diet now more than ever. So, let's talk!

Olive oil

The mainstay of the Mediterranean diet is olive oil. Forty years ago, when the original studies were published describing the health effects of the Mediterranean diet, they described a diet high in fat. What's important to point out, though, is that olive oil is the principal source of this fat. The olive tree is native to the Mediterranean basin and there is archaeological evidence that humans collected wild olives as far back as 8000 BCE and began turning olives into olive oil as far back as 6000 BCE. There is also evidence of commercial milling of olive oil in Egypt, Palestine, Lebanon, and Israel as far back as 1000 BCE.

These days, worldwide production of olive oil is around 3 million tonnes annually. Spain is by far the world's biggest producer (1,781,000 tonnes), followed by Italy (463,000 tonnes).

Olive oil production

After olives are picked from the tree, they are crushed (or pressed) into an olive paste. The paste is mixed (called malaxed) to allow the microscopic oil droplets in the paste to stick together. The oil is then separated from the watery matter and fruit pulp with the use of a press (the traditional method) or centrifugation (the modern method). This process is simple and natural. And that's quite a contrast to many of the modern vegetable oils which undergo complex chemical processes.

Virgin olive oils are the oils made from the first pressing of the olives, which removes about 90% of the olives' juice. Virgin olive oils are produced using mechanical means only, with no chemical or heat treatment allowed after the pressing process. Within the umbrella term of virgin olive oil there are several sub-categories.

The differences between the various virgin olive oils primarily relate to the amount of acid in the oil.

Getting the good oil

- Premium extra-virgin olive oil – this is the finest oil. It has extremely low acidity (as low as 0.225%) and is best used in uncooked dishes where you can appreciate its flavours, colour and aroma.
- Extra-virgin olive oil (EVOO) – this oil can vary in colour from pale yellow to green. According to international olive oil council regulations, extra-virgin olive oil is no more than 0.8% acidity. Like premium extra-virgin olive oil, this is best uncooked so you can appreciate its flavours.
- Virgin olive oil – with an acid content up to 2%, it is generally thought to be good for cooking but still with enough flavour to enjoy uncooked.
- Pure olive oil (or olive oil) – is lower quality and sent to a processing plant and refined using heat, chemicals or filtration. Post-processing, the oil is clear, odourless and flavourless but has a long shelf-life, which is a major attraction. Olive oils which have been refined are called 'pure olive oil' and are best for cooking.
- Light and lite olive oil (sometimes called mild olive oil) – have undergone a filtration process to remove much of the natural colour and flavour. These oils are often used in cooking or baking where the fruity flavour of extra-virgin olive oil isn't needed. With these oils, 'light' doesn't mean low in calories, but rather low in flavour. The calorie content of these oils is the same as any other olive oil. The term 'light' can also be used alongside the terms extra-virgin olive oil and virgin olive oil.

The colour of oil

Olive oils are generally pale yellow or green. The green oils come from unripe olives and generally impart a slightly bitter, pungent flavour. Golden or yellow coloured oils are olive oils prepared from ripe olives. These oils have a smoother, more buttery taste without the bitterness, and are perfect for adding to subtly-flavoured foods.

Fried it is

Conventional wisdom says that fried food is bad for us. But this is not necessarily true. It depends, very much, on which oil food is fried in. The evidence suggests food fried in extra virgin olive oil (EVOO) may even impart positive nutritional value. A Spanish team of scientists[37] cooked eggplant, tomato, pumpkin and potato. They compared 3 methods: frying using EVOO, boiling, and cooking using a mix of EVOO and water. Using highly specialised equipment, the team measured the levels of health promoting polyphenols in the foods. As it turns out, frying in EVOO is the most effective way to increase the polyphenolic and anti-oxidant content of food. Frying in EVOO increased the polyphenolic content of the vegetables. This doesn't mean all fried food is good. It is unlikely that the fish and chips you buy from the local shop are cooked in EVOO. Hence, this finding does nothing to change the general premise that takeaway fried food is an 'only occasional' food. But this study has important implications when it comes to your home cooking. Using a high-quality olive oil will enhance the health benefits of your meal rather than detract from it. Put simply, frying foods isn't necessarily bad. The evidence we have is that foods fried in olive oil are associated with net positive health effects.

Large studies that have explored the association between a diet high in foods fried in olive oil and health outcomes report a reduction in the risk of many of the metabolic syndrome complications. Specifically, a reduction in the risk of heart disease and high blood pressure.[36] Cooking with olive oil promotes the release of many of the health-promoting chemicals from vegetables. The more olive oil used in cooking and the greater the cooking time are associated with larger releases of health-promoting antioxidants and polyphenols.[37] Heating olive oil does not destroy its health-giving qualities. If cost is not an issue, then frying in EVOO is likely to have greater health benefits than the cheaper olive oils.

Which olive oil should I choose?

Virgin olive oil is believed to possess the greatest health benefits as it retains most of the nutrients from the olive fruit. In addition, locally produced oils may have additional benefits over imported oils because of the potential breakdown in vital nutrients that can occur with prolonged storage. I don't mean to say you should be using expensive, locally produced extra-virgin olive oil as your only oil. Cost by itself doesn't necessarily correlate with health benefits. What I am suggesting is that there are significant health benefits for your liver and general health when using olive oil as your predominant source of dietary fat. Using EVOO with breads and salads, and virgin olive oil or olive oil for cooking is strongly recommended. The more olive oil you have in your diet the better, you can't overdo it.

Use olive oil as the primary oil for all culinary and cooking needs.

Fruit, vegetables and grains

In almost all dietary advice, a diet high in fruit and vegetables is recommended. In the typical Mediterranean diet, plant-based foods constitute the core of the diet with animal-based foods eaten only occasionally. All fruits and vegetables are good for you. That fact is simple and difficult to argue. And the more you have, the greater the health benefits.

Exactly how fruit and vegetables exert their beneficial health effects is still debated. Diets high in grains, fruits and vegetables lead to reduction in blood measures of inflammation. Inflammation is bad for us, driving our metabolism towards insulin resistance. The mechanism for this reduction in inflammation comes from changes in our gut flora.[38]

Fruit or veggies – does it matter?

Is it reasonable that fruit and vegetables are lumped together in discussions of what's best to eat for optimal liver health? I'm well into my 50's, and up until recently, wasn't sure what the difference was between a fruit and a vegetable. Of course, I knew a carrot was a vegetable and so was a potato, and that apples and pears were fruit. Okay, but what is a tomato? What is a pumpkin? Peas? Well, believe it or not, tomatoes, pumpkins and peas are all fruit. Fruit is defined as a seed-bearing structure that develops from a flowing plant; and vegetables are all the other plant parts such as roots, leaves and stems.

The Australian Government Guidelines (NHMRC) on healthy fruit and vegetable intake recommend 5 serves of vegetables daily (375 g) and 2 serves of fruit. When it comes to fatty liver disease fruit and vegetables both exert similar, positive health benefits. The more fruit you have, the lower the risk of fatty liver disease, and the same is true for vegetables.[39]

Get your reds . . . and purple and blue vegetables

I was walking with my son one evening and we got involved in a meandering conversation, which included the fact that cats and dogs don't see colours in the same way as humans do. Humans see yellow, orange and red as distinct colours; whereas cats and dogs see less distinct, pale grey versions. It dawned on me that this difference in colour vision might have some evolutionary explanation.

One of the theories for why humans and other primates have evolved to see these colours better than other mammalian species, is that it allows us to identify fruit and vegetables in nature more easily, and therefore offers us a survival advantage. But not all fruit and vegetables are yellow, orange or red. Plenty are white or green. But is there anything special about vegetables coloured at the red or yellow end of the spectrum that offers us a particular survival advantage? Are red, orange and yellow fruits and vegetables any different from white and green vegetables? The answer is yes.

Yellow, red, orange and blue fruit and vegetables are pigmented by a group of compounds called anthocyanins. Anthocyanins form one of the principle pigments in these brightly coloured foods, and are a type of polyphenol. I discussed polyphenols earlier: they are a group of plant-based chemicals associated with protection from fatty liver disease and other components of metabolic syndrome. Anthocyanins are usually present in the skins of these fruits and vegetables and their concentration varies markedly – usually reflected in the colour intensity of these foods.

Now, what we really want to know is whether these brightly pigmented foods offer any particular advantage when it comes to liver health, or health in general. The one human study we have comes from the Department of Nutrition, in Shaoguan, China. In this study, 72 overweight Chinese men and women with fatty liver disease were divided into 2 groups.[40] One group received purified anthocyanin derived from bilberry and blackcurrant; the other half received a placebo. The study went for just 3 months, and measured liver function and insulin resistance in both groups at the start and end of the 3 months. Those taking the anthocyanin supplement experienced significant improvement in their liver function tests during the study period – and their insulin resistance improved too. The liver function tests and insulin resistance measures of those taking the placebo didn't change. Weight didn't change in either group.

Again, the observation that weight remained unchanged, but liver function improved, is crucially important. At the risk of repeating myself, I will drag you through what these facts mean to me. Fatty liver is perhaps the most common clinical manifestation of metabolic syndrome/insulin resistance. Apart from the direct liver injury it causes, it is also a potent marker of future risk of diabetes, heart disease, stroke and cancer. Importantly it is reversible. The point I wish to emphasise here is that improvement in liver health and metabolic health can be independent of any change in weight. Change in diet can change your metabolism for the better even if you don't lose weight.

Top 10 common foods containing high levels of anthocyanins

1 Purple corn
2 Eggplant
3 Blackberries
4 Blueberries
5 Red currants
6 Black currants
7 Blood orange
8 Cherries
9 Plums
10 Kidney beans

Interestingly, high concentrations of anthocyanins are also present in red wine and almost all berries. Given that the mechanisms causing diabetes (as well as cardiovascular disease and many cancers) and fatty liver disease are essentially the same, studies showing the benefits of berries in reducing the risk of developing diabetes are relevant too. A large study from Harvard Medical School, Boston[41], pooled data from 3 previous smaller surveys. The study aimed to explore the dietary components associated with the prevention of the development of future diabetes. The study collected data from 200,000 people who were free from diabetes at baseline. Patients were then followed and re-interviewed every second year over a number of years. With more than 3.5 million person-years of follow-up data available for analysis, the magnitude of the study was enormous. What the study reported was that higher rates of anthocyanin intake were associated with a reduced risk of developing diabetes. This was true even after the results were adjusted for other factors that may contribute to diabetes risk such as age, BMI, lifestyle and dietary factors.

Carrots – good for your eyes and good for your liver

That line your mother fed you, that if you ate all your carrots you would have perfect eyesight, is based in fact. Carrots contain large amounts of a chemical called beta-carotene, which is converted into vitamin A in the body. Vitamin A is necessary for retinal health, especially for good low-light vision. One of the first symptoms people with a deficiency in vitamin A notice is loss of night-time or low-light vision. Vitamin A is also necessary for the healthy development of the retina in babies, with vitamin A deficiency the most common cause of blindness in children worldwide. So, your mum was right!

Medicine is interesting for lots of reasons, and one of them is the people. Person-to-person contact keeps medicine alive, from the doctor/patient relationship to interactions between colleagues and junior doctors-in-training. I was in the middle of training a junior doctor on gastroscopies one day, when she told me a remarkable tale related to her personal health. She described that as a medical student at university, she noticed herself slowly turning yellow. First, the palms of her hands had appeared a little yellow, and then over the next week or 2, people started to comment that her facial skin had taken on a yellow hue.

Now, when it comes to their own health, there are 2 types of doctors – the neurotics and the blasé. Most of us start off in the neurotic camp, where we believe every little symptom we experience is the manifestation of a rare and incurable disease, and over the years become more blasé, head in the sand types who feel themselves indestructible. So, my junior colleague told me of her distress as she self-diagnosed a case of progressive jaundice, one of the first symptoms of liver failure.

But as it turned out, there was more to the story. My colleague described the fad diet she was on at the time – all she ate was carrots. Numerous tests identified that her evolving yellow complexion wasn't a sign of progressive liver disease, but a reflection of too many carrots in her diet. She had developed carotenaemia.

Beta-carotene is the pigment that gives carrots and other red foods – and some medical students – their colour. Beta-carotene is a precursor that your body turns into vitamin A. Beta-carotene also has potent anti-inflammatory and antioxidant effects. Importantly, the higher the concentration of beta-carotene in your blood, the lower your risk of liver disease.[42,43] The link between blood levels and health isn't just specific to liver disease. Dr Jun Liu from the School of Public Health, Guizhou, China explored the hypothesis that these compounds may not just protect individuals from fatty liver, but from all aspects of metabolic syndrome.[44] Using data from more than 2,000 middle-aged Chinese men and women they demonstrated that the higher the concentration of beta-carotene in your blood the lower your risk of obesity, diabetes and high cholesterol.

Ten foods high in beta-carotene

1. Sweet potato
2. Carrots
3. Spinach
4. Cos lettuce
5. Butternut squash
6. Cantaloupe
7. Sweet red pepper
8. Dried apricots
9. Peas
10. Broccoli

Nuts

Nuts are good for you. This should come as no surprise. Put simply, anything made and packaged by nature is beneficial for liver health. Nuts are no exception. Full of healthy mono-unsaturated fats, nuts are high in fibre and have few or no carbohydrates. They are high in important trace elements such as calcium, manganese, magnesium, selenium and a variety of antioxidants. Nuts are also a potent appetite suppressant and great as a snack or meal alternative. Evidence suggests that the more nuts you consume, the lower your liver fat.[45] Eating nuts is also associated with general health benefits such a reducing the risk of heart disease and diabetes.

Our medical colleagues in Barcelona also provide compelling information about the long-term health benefits of nuts. In the PREDIMED trial (which I will discuss in detail in the following pages) patients had their diet supplemented with either extra-virgin olive oil or nuts. After 6 years in the trial, both groups had reductions in liver fat.[46] Those in the nut group also lost weight over time compared to patients on a standard diet. There are not many interventions that result in people losing weight over this sort of timeline. So although nuts are calorie-dense, they do not appear to be associated with weight gain. Great news!

Fibre

Dietary fibre, also called roughage, is the non-digestible portion of plant-based foods. It goes in one end and most of it comes out the other. There are numerous compounds that make up dietary fibre, including cellulose, pectins and fructans. The scientific world divides fibre into 2 main components: water soluble fibre and insoluble fibre. Soluble fibre is beneficial for microbiome health. After digestion in the small bowel, the dissolved fibre particles are rapidly transported to the colon where the vast majority of bowel organisms reside. Here, the bacteria feast on the fibre, generating gases and a number of metabolically active by-products. These bacterial-generated chemicals include short chain fatty acids, butyrate and propionate. Butyrate is now well recognised as having beneficial effects on the health of the colon and may protect against colonic cancer. Common examples of foods high in soluble fibre include: black beans, avocados, broccoli, pears and apples.

Ten foods high in soluble fibre

1 Brussels sprouts
2 Barley
3 Flaxseeds
4 Lima beans
5 Sweet potato
6 Turnips
7 Kidney beans
8 Figs
9 Nectarines
10 Carrots

Insoluble fibre primarily provides bulk to the stool and also draws in water to the stool aiding defecation. Insoluble fibre is more resistant to digestion by colonic bacteria than soluble fibre, but small amounts are fermented. Common foods high in insoluble fibre include bran, nuts, leafy vegetables and seeds.

Fibre bulks up food and may reduce its palatability, and both of these are associated with eating less. Fibre in food also draws water into it, contributing to gastric distension, reducing appetite and increasing satiety. This helps explain why a diet high in fibre contributes to protection from obesity.

It is estimated that our Palaeolithic ancestors' daily fibre intake was in the order of 80–120 g.[47] Current nutritional guidelines recommend 30 g of dietary fibre daily for men and 25 g daily for women. In Australia, less than 30% of adults currently consume that much fibre.[48] Low fibre intake has been linked to adverse clinical outcomes including bowel cancer, diabetes, obesity, heart disease, haemorrhoids, diverticular disease and, of course, liver disease.

Low fibre intake is very common in people with fatty liver disease. One detailed study explored the dietary fibre intake of 50 people. Half had fatty liver and the other half had healthy liver function. The individuals were matched for age, sex and BMI. The daily fibre intake of those with healthy livers was nearly twice that of those with fatty liver disease (23 g compared with 13 g).[49] Other studies have revealed a close inverse relationship between the amount of fibre in the diet and liver fat on MRI.[50] At present, there is only one interventional study that has explored the potential role of additional dietary fibre as a treatment for fatty liver.

This one small study reveals how potentially effective, simple, cheap dietary interventions can be for liver health. The study was run by Dr Daubioul and colleagues from the Université Catholique de Lovain in Brussels. It involved just 7 patients who had previously been diagnosed with fatty liver disease. Each participant received 16 g of supplemental fibre in their daily diet for 8 weeks. Liver function and insulin levels were compared before and after the fibre supplement. Both liver function and insulin levels improved during the course of the study.[51]

Fibre, by definition, is not absorbed across the intestinal membrane. Any beneficial effect it has on liver health is enacted via its impact on gut flora. Our gut flora is its own biosphere. It is made up of billions of bugs. Keeping this ecosystem healthy with a diet high in fibre is central to ensuring our liver health and our health more generally. Soluble fibre acts as the natural fertiliser for our gut flora, and is food for our gut bacteria, aiding bacteria proliferation and supporting healthy diversity in the microbiome.

Another way fibre keeps us all healthy is by preventing leaky gut. Leaky gut is where the toxic, inflammatory chemicals synthesised in the bowel by unhealthy flora are absorbed directly into the blood across a porous gut lining. These chemicals then travel up to the liver causing liver damage. Fibre feeds the healthy gut bugs, reducing production of these pathogenic chemicals and preventing leaky gut and associated liver damage.[52]

Foods and their amounts of fibre

Food	Serving	Soluble fibre (g)	Insoluble fibre (g)	Total fibre (g)
Apple	1 medium	4.2	1.5	5.7
Banana	1 medium	1.8	1.7	3.5
Strawberry	1 cup	1.8	2.6	4.4
Almonds	1 ounce	0.7	3.5	4.2
Peanuts	1 ounce	1.1	1.2	2.3
Broccoli	1 cup	1.3	1.4	2.7
Carrot	1 medium	1.1	1.5	2.6
Potato (with skin)	1 medium	2.4	2.4	4.8
Quinoa (cooked)	1 cup	3.4	5.0	8.4
Rye bread	1 slice	1.9	0.8	2.7
Wholegrain bread	1 slice	2.8	0.1	2.9

Fish and seafood

The traditional Mediterranean diet is high in fish and other seafood and low in red meat. Some fish contain high concentrations of a fat called omega-3 fatty acid. Consumption of this fat is strongly associated with reduced levels of inflammation in the blood and liver. Omega-3 fatty acids cannot be synthesised by the human body and therefore need to be obtained through the diet. Fish, however, can synthesise omega-3 fatty acid from the ingestion of seaweed and other sea plants. Some fish species store large amounts of omega-3 fatty acid in their flesh and diets high in these species have been associated with the greatest health benefits.

Fish rich in omega-3 include trout, tuna, salmon, mackerel and sardines; whereas sole, snapper and flounder contain hardly any. However numerous studies show a diet high in fish (without specifying what type) lowers your risk of death from liver disease and also reduces the risk of developing liver cancer.[53,54] There is actually little science that explores whether liver health benefits from a diet high in omega-3 fatty acid–rich fish compared with other species. The science we do have suggests that the more fish in your diet, the better for your general health. My suggestion is to eat whatever type of fish you prefer. In Chapter 8, I discuss the science behind omega-3 fatty acid supplements and liver health. But simply, when it comes to fish in the diet, the more the merrier. It's good for liver health.

Chicken

Chicken just isn't sexy enough – there is almost no dietary science exploring whether a diet high or low in poultry is good or bad for liver health. One of the few studies we do have explored the issue of meat consumption generally and the risk of liver cancer. Liver cancer is a really interesting and powerful end point because it almost always occurs after years of liver damage, most frequently from fatty liver. Dietary components that may have an effect on liver health are thought to either increase or reduce the development of liver cancer.

A meta-analysis is a study whereby the data from a large number of smaller studies exploring a particular topic is pooled. Dr Luo and colleagues from the Zhejiang Cancer Hospital in Hangzhou, China undertook one such study exploring dietary sources of meat and the subsequent development of liver cancer.[54] They found that the more poultry in your diet, the lower your risk of liver cancer. The authors reported that poultry and fish appeared to offer similar degrees of protection from liver cancer. Interestingly, both are integral components of the Mediterranean diet.

A second study offers similarly reassuring data on dietary poultry and liver health. Published by the Division of Cancer Epidemiology and Genetics, Rockville USA, the authors used dietary information from half a million men and women who had completed a food questionnaire in the mid-1990s.[55] In the mid-2000s, the researchers looked at the causes of death of people in the study who had died, and examined the data for any potential associations. They found that those whose diets were high in poultry had a 30% lower risk of liver cancer and death from cirrhosis compared with those who ate little poultry. This data adds to my confidence that the association is real.

Red meat

A common belief is that red meat is bad for your liver. When I chat with patients about diet and liver disease, they often suggest that red meat is 'hard to digest and puts a strain' on the liver. The implication being that if you can make the liver work less hard it will result in improved liver health . . . Well this, like many urban myths is, probably, partly true. Red meat (lamb, beef and pork) forms only a minor component of the Mediterranean diet. Although there is no scientific evidence that the liver works 'harder' after a meal containing red meat, there is some data suggesting a diet high in red meat may have detrimental effects on liver health. But it's not black and white.[55,56]

The last few decades have seen world red meat consumption increase. At the same time the evidence tying red meat consumption with the development of liver disease, insulin resistance, diabetes and heart disease is becoming more widely accepted. If you wish to maintain liver health, regular consumption of red meats or processed meats should be avoided. The more of the meats you have, the worse it is for you. It is also not just the quantity of meat consumed, but also the way it is cooked that impacts liver health. What is emerging is that grilling or frying meats for a prolonged time (to 'well done') is associated with the development of liver damaging compounds. There are 2 classes of compounds generated when cooking meats these ways:[57] advanced glycosylation end products (AGEs) and heterotrophic amines (HCAs).

Both are associated with the progression of fatty liver disease, diabetes and cancer.[58]

Red meat is highly nutritious and full of vitamins and minerals. So, while red meat doesn't need to be totally avoided, fish should be your first choice because of its special metabolic benefits in reducing inflammation and improving blood clotting. Poultry, as we have just discussed, is an acceptable healthy alternative to fish. In the Mediterranean diet, red meat is eaten just a few times a month in small quantities. My advice would be to have red meat as an occasional food only.

Fat

I don't think there is any word in the sphere of health or nutrition more evocative than 'fat'. In our current culture, the word suggests ill health, laziness, poor food choices and, perhaps, even ugliness. It appears logical, of course, that eating fatty food is the culprit and should be avoided. Even more so, it would seem apparent that to facilitate liver health you should avoid fat. After all, fatty liver is one of the commonest liver conditions in the world; liver fat causes scarring and liver damage and can result in cirrhosis. At face value this all appears quite logical. The problem with this stream of thought is that it is wrong.

Let's talk through these associations and try to separate *fat* from fiction. The first thing to emphasise about body fat is that it is essential for our existence. Fat is a vital part of the physical makeup of all humans. It is in every cell of the body and it makes up about 60% of the brain. As well as the fat in our individual cells, the body stores fat – adipose tissue – in the chest, abdomen and beneath the skin. The normal amount of adipose tissues varies between the sexes and with age. In a healthy 25-year-old woman, body fat is about 25% of total weight and about 17% in a man of the same age. This percentage increases in both women and men as they age. This physiological fat forms multiple functions: it protects the organs from physical damage; it insulates us from heat and cold; it stores calories; and fat is needed to synthesize multiple hormones essential for health.

Excess body fat can also be the consequence of choosing foods with a negative impact on body metabolism. However, eating foods that contain fat doesn't necessarily mean more fat in your body. Or we could say it like this: just as eating meat (muscle) doesn't result in muscle growth, eating fat doesn't automatically result in you getting fatter.

Why include fat?

Fat makes many foods taste better. But there are also many solid health reasons to get adequate amounts of healthy fat in your diet. What's important to understand though, is that not all fats are the same – there are good fats and bad fats.

Unsaturated fats are generally the good fats. These fats reduce inflammation, lower cholesterol levels and reduce liver fat. There are 2 types of unsaturated fat:

Monounsaturated fats are found in:

- olive oil
- nuts (almonds, peanuts, pecans)
- avocado
- seeds.

Polyunsaturated fats are found in:

- fish
- nuts (walnuts)
- sunflower seeds.

Omega-3 fats are a type of polyunsaturated fat that cannot be synthesised by the body. These fats must be obtained from the diet. Good sources of these fats include fish, nuts, seeds, and fish oil supplements.

Saturated fats have historically been considered to be the bad fats. Over more recent years this conclusion appears less straightforward. Saturated fats are found in animal-based foods such as beef, cheese, ice cream, and in coconut oil and palm oil.

Saturated fats are found in:

- red meat
- dairy
- coconut oil
- palm oil.

It may seem remarkable that coconut oil appears on the list of foods containing high concentrations of bad saturated fats. In the media, coconut oil has been touted for its health benefits. But promotion online or elsewhere isn't necessarily supported by science. You might have heard or read that populations consuming substantial amounts of coconut have few symptoms of metabolic syndrome. However, these Indigenous populations are consuming either coconut flesh or coconut cream, which is metabolically quite different from the refined oil.

Diets supplemented with significant quantities of coconut oil are almost certainly bad for us. When part of a high calorie diet, coconut oil is associated with dramatic increases in liver fat and exacerbation of insulin resistance. It may be much worse metabolically than a diet high in sugar – which we know is poison.[59] There are no long-term studies exploring the relationship between a diet supplemented with coconut oil and the complications of metabolic syndrome. The studies we do have suggest that coconut oil has a negative effect on cholesterol profiles, increasing the levels of the bad LDL-cholesterol.[60] The evidence suggests that coconut oil should be viewed the same as other sources of bad saturated fats, which we will discuss in the following pages.

The good 'uns

The most studied source of unsaturated fat is olive oil. And all the evidence says that the more you consume the better it is for your liver health. Olive oil reduces liver fat, liver scarring and liver cancer risk. However, this association isn't just true for olive oil, but appears to be true for all sources of unsaturated fat.

Although obesity is less frequent in India than in many Western counties, other aspects of metabolic syndrome are surprisingly common. The cause, or causes, of this is still a matter of debate, but it is likely that the cooking oil choices in India are part of the problem as they are typically high in saturated fat, such as soya bean or safflower oil. Interestingly, Indians often develop fatty liver disease and other aspects of metabolic syndrome at a much lower weight than their Caucasian counterparts.

Doctors Nigam and Pasha from the National Diabetes, Obesity and Cholesterol Foundation in New Delhi, India, explored whether changing the cooking oil from a standard oil, high in saturated fat (safflower or soybean), to olive or canola oil (canola oil is high in unsaturated fat) was beneficial for people with fatty liver disease. They found that changing cooking oil significantly improved liver heath by markedly reducing liver fat in those who moved to either olive oil or canola oil. Although the improvement in liver health was expected, there were other dramatic changes observed during the study period: despite the total calorie intake being constant across all study participants, irrespective of the cooking oil they were using, those who changed to olive oil lost 5 kg in weight during the 6 months of the study. Those who changed to canola oil, lost 4 kg. But those who stayed with saturated fat cooking oil lost no weight. Insulin levels also fell enormously in the 2 groups that changed to cooking with unsaturated fat oils.[61]

These results weren't just a flash in the pan, they have been replicated by other studies.[62] In addition, the health benefits of unsaturated fats don't just apply to fatty liver and weight loss, but also include reduced liver cancer risk.[63] It seems paradoxical to suggest, but the more fat in the diet, the lower the risk of liver fat and liver damage. It's true! Of course, the caveat is to use only unsaturated fat.

The PREDIMED trial

In 2003 Spanish researchers initiated an enormous study to scientifically explore whether the Mediterranean diet improves health.[46] This study was titled (in Spanish) *Prevención con Dieta Mediterránea*, shortened to the PREDIMED trial. Up until the PREDIMED trial, most of the health outcomes relating to the Mediterranean diet were from small, prospective studies or those that reported association (of the diet with a particular positive health outcome) and therefore could not prove causation. PREDIMED stands for primary prevention of cardiovascular disease with a Mediterranean diet. The researchers enrolled more than 7,000 Spaniards with various complications of metabolic syndrome who were all at high risk of heart disease. The participants were randomly assigned to one of 3 dietary interventions: a Mediterranean diet supplemented with extra-virgin olive oil (EVOO), a Mediterranean diet supplemented with nuts (which are high in unsaturated fats), or a standard low-fat diet, which served as the control group.

Participants in the Mediterranean arms of the study received either one litre of EVOO or 210 g of nuts each week, donated by local producers. All were given support and advice to help them adhere to the diets. The aim was to follow participants over many years to see whether the Mediterranean diet offered a reduction in the risk of heart attack and stroke (both consequences of insulin resistance).

In 2013, well before the study was due to conclude, the researchers were contacted by the Safety Committee and told to stop the project immediately. A safety committee is an independent group of clinicians whose role is to examine the trial data throughout the project and make sure no harm comes to patients. What the committee had found by 2013 was that both the oil and nut arms of the study were associated with such marked reductions in heart attack and stroke, compared with the group on the standard low-fat diet, that it was unsafe for individuals to continue on this low-fat diet.

Apart from a marked reduction in heart attack and stroke, the Mediterranean diet was associated with protection against memory loss, diabetes, breast cancer, high cholesterol and high blood pressure (unfortunately liver function was not examined in this study). It may be expected that those on the high-fat Mediterranean diet would gain weight, but they actually lost weight.

The dietary advice that has been drummed into most of us over the last 2 decades is to consume fruit and vegetables but avoid fat. This was the advice offered to the control group within the study. Unfortunately, this diet group experienced a 30% higher risk of heart attack and stroke compared to the high-fat Mediterranean diets. The PREDIMED trial demonstrated that the current dietary guidelines in many countries may actually be causing harm and contributing to disease. This counter-intuitive message, that a high-fat diet protects from heart attack, stroke, diabetes, memory loss, cancer and weight gain is one of the core messages of *Liver Better Life*. The smoking gun!

Let's boil it down

- Fat makes up about 25% of our body composition.
- Fatty tissue in the body is essential for health.
- Dietary fat isn't directly converted into body fat.
- Some fat in the diet is essential for health.
- Unsaturated fats are good for liver health.
- Omega-3 is essential for health, and must be obtained from our diets.

Dairy, yoghurt and good bacteria

Dairy products are a small but intrinsic part of the Mediterranean diet and therefore are recommended in *Liver Better Life*. Although dairy contains saturated fat, it is full of hundreds of other proteins, sugars and trace elements. There is currently no dairy-specific liver health benefits or liabilities in the scientific literature.[64,65] There are 2 small studies that explore whether yoghurt may offer beneficial liver health effects.[66,67] Complicating the picture slightly was the fact that both studies used a probiotic yoghurt. The results were positive, indicating a reduction in liver fat. Due to the design of the studies however, it is not possible to determine whether the positive effect was from the yoghurt or the probiotic. As we discussed much earlier, probiotics result in decreased liver fat. So, at present, feel free to consume dairy (especially probiotic yoghurt) regularly and enjoy it.

Chocolate love

In our modern world, we are spoilt for choice in almost all aspects of our life. Food is no exception. There is an almost infinite range of foods available at any one place and time. Yet even given this incredible choice, chocolate still holds a special place in the lives of many people as a unique food.

The origin of chocolate

Chocolate was first consumed by the ancient civilisations of Central America nearly 4 millennia ago. The Aztecs made chocolate drinks from the seeds of the cacao tree. Introduced to Europe by the Spanish, chocolate was consumed as a drink mixed with honey or sugar to overcome the naturally bitter flavour. It wasn't until the 1800s that chocolate in its current solid form was first developed. Milk chocolate was developed by mixing chocolate liquor with powdered milk by Henri Nestlé of the Nestlé Empire in 1875.

Despite originating in Central America, most chocolate consumed today is derived from cocoa grown in Western Africa and Indonesia. Chocolate comes from the cacao tree, which produces large fruits (pods) that contain between 20 and 50 cocoa beans. The cacao tree flowers and bears fruit throughout the entire year. These pods are harvested by hand using either machetes or sticks. The annual crop from one tree is only about half a kilogram of cocoa. The seeds of the cacao tree are naturally very bitter and must be fermented to release the unique flavour we are familiar with. After fermentation the beans are cleaned, dried and roasted. The raw cocoa in this form may be ground into cocoa mass. The cocoa mass is liquefied by heating – at this stage it is called, cocoa liquor. The liquor is then cooled and then separated into cocoa solids and cocoa butter. It is from these 2 basic components that the commercial chocolate we consume today is produced.

Dark chocolate is a mix of cocoa butter and solids, sugar, cocoa liquor and sometimes vanilla; while milk chocolate/white chocolate is cocoa butter, sugar, cocoa liquor and milk powder, and sometimes vanilla.

Chocolate and liver health

Reports of chocolate having medicinal benefits date back to the times of the Aztecs and Mayans. Modern scientific studies have been conducted on the effects of chocolate on the cardiovascular system, skin, brain and most importantly, of course, the liver. Put simply, chocolate reduces liver fat and inflammation, the basic pathological mechanisms that drive liver disease from all causes. Chocolate also appears to reduce insulin levels. The more often you consume chocolate, the greater the beneficial effect on liver health. In clinical studies, individuals who had the best parameters of liver health were those consuming chocolate every day.[68]

Chocolate's health benefits are not just confined to the liver. It is well established that chocolate also exerts a positive impact on cardiovascular health, blood pressure and cholesterol levels. While it may come as a surprise, chocolate is just the refined fruit of the cacao tree; a perfectly natural, complex food full of numerous different natural chemicals that do you good – however it does have some added sugar.

Chocolate contains large amounts of polyphenols, as do fruit and vegetables, wine, olive oil and coffee – many of the foods that form the basis of *Liver Better Life*. As polyphenols are present in almost all liver fortifying foods, it doesn't take a great leap to ask whether it is the polyphenol content of these foods that creates the liver health benefits. The answer at present though, is we don't know! There are only a few small studies on the use of polyphenol supplements for liver disease. Although they suggest there may be a benefit, the data is too limited as yet to be recommending these supplements routinely.[69]

As there are literally thousands of different polyphenols in our foods, I think the potential health benefits of these compounds are unlikely to come from supplementation into our diets of just one or 2 different polyphenols. More likely, the health benefits relate to the complex mix of hundreds of compounds together, rather than the individual compounds per se. As with vitamin supplements, while vitamins are essential for our health, the wholefood that contains the vitamin is much greater than a vitamin supplement when it comes to health generally and liver health specifically.

Chocolate makes your liver healthier and your brain smarter

Chocolate, like coffee, is one of those fascinating foods that appear to have positive and widespread metabolic effects on a variety of organ systems, including the brain. The evidence suggests that chocolate reduces cognitive decline in older people,[70] indicating a potential role in reducing the risk of developing Alzheimer's disease or in delaying its development. Other studies have shown regular chocolate eating may improve cognitive function in elderly people who already display some deficits,[71] and can improve cognitive function in elderly people who were cognitively well.[72]

The intellectual benefits of chocolate aren't just for the elderly. One study measured a variety of cognitive parameters in 20-year-olds after they drank a glass of chocolate milk. The study found significant improvement in protection from mental fatigue,[73] with benefits demonstrated as early as 10 minutes after the drink. Other studies have revealed even more widespread improvements in cognitive function after eating chocolate.[74]

It is thought that chocolate affects the brain via 2 distinct mechanisms. It relaxes the blood vessels, increasing blood flow, and also acts directly on brain cells to increase expression of chemicals that protect the brain from injury and promote brain cell growth.[75]

Franz Messerli, a physician from New York,[76] performed one of the most interesting studies I've ever read. Exploring the hypothesis that chocolate makes you smarter, he looked at the relationship between chocolate consumption on a per capita level and Nobel Prizes awarded to the citizens of that country. He used the number of Nobel Laureates as a marker of a country's overall cognitive function, or how smart each country's citizens were.

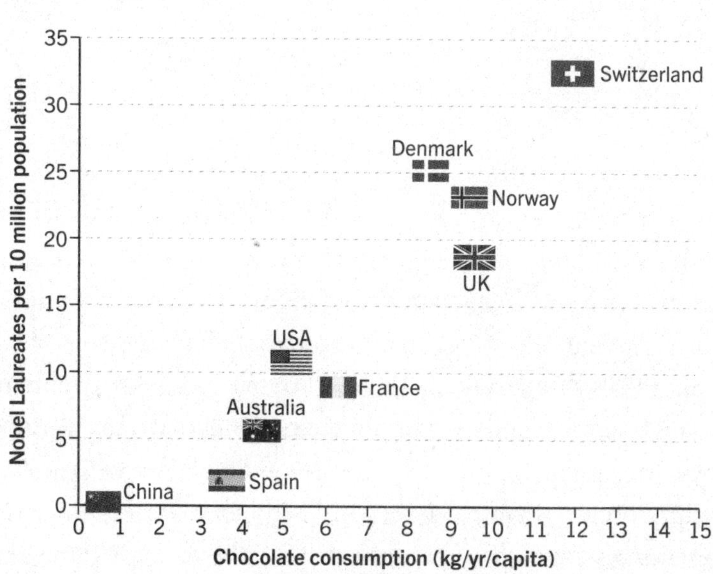

Figure 5.2 The relationship between chocolate consumption and number of Nobel Prizes awarded.

Dr Messerli found a surprisingly close correlation between the 2 parameters. The Swiss were the clear winners, with the most Nobel Laureates per capita and the greatest chocolate consumption, at a remarkable 12 kg per person per year. At the other end of the scale were China, Japan, and Portugal – who clearly need to eat more chocolate. Australia was disappointing too, eating only 4.5 kg per person per year, which is about one third of the average Swiss intake and with a Nobel Laureate rate of one sixth that of the Swiss.

World's biggest chocolate consumers[77]

1 Switzerland
2 Germany
3 Ireland
4 United Kingdom
5 Norway
6 Sweden
7 Australia
8 Netherlands
9 United States
10 France

But chocolate affects more than cognition – it has demonstrable effects on mood too. In 1993, Weisenberg and colleagues from the BarHan University, Israel, examined whether chocolate consumption could negate negative emotions. To induce negative emotions,[78] the authors asked the study participants to attempt to solve an unsolvable problem. The researchers knew the problem was unsolvable but, of course, the participants didn't. The unsolvable task was designed to induce feelings of helplessness and anxiety. The experiment involved 4 sets of cards that varied by 4 different parameters, which were dealt out to the subjects who had to identify the pattern. Of course, there was no pattern to identify. At the end of this initial phase, participants were asked to complete an assessment measuring their anxiety level. Sounds cruel, doesn't it? And where does chocolate fit into the psychologists' mind games?

At the end of the first round, participants were given 50 g of chocolate and the experiment was repeated. After consuming the chocolate, levels of anxiety fell significantly. Although not all studies examining chocolate and cognitive performance are positive, the clear balance of the literature suggests that chocolate consumption, both in the short and long terms and in the young and elderly, is associated with positive outcomes.

Chocolate and heart health

On the sun-drenched San Blas Islands of Panama live the Indigenous Kuna people. This was the first population in the world recognised as having blood pressure that didn't rise as people aged.[79] A series of studies performed over many years by Norman Hollenberg and colleagues from the Brigham and Women's Hospital in Boston demonstrated that this phenomenon was somehow related to the Kuna's diet. When members of the communities moved from the local islands to the mainland, and their diet changed, their blood pressure increased. This link with moving to the mainland essentially meant that there was some protective environmental explanation associated with living on the islands and indicated that genetic causes were unlikely.

Dr Hollenberg also wondered whether their low blood pressure protected the locals from dying from blood pressure-related disease such as heart attack and stroke. On examining death records, he found something truly astounding: the Kuna people living on their local island and consuming their indigenous diet had a death rate from cardiovascular disease of 9.2 deaths per 100,000 people. This contrasts with 83.4 deaths per 100,000 people when this population moved to the mainland.

The component of the diet that made this population unique from all others was their consumption of cocoa (cocoa are the seeds from which chocolate is made). The Islander Kuna people drank locally grown cocoa as their major source of fluid.[80] This locally grown cocoa was high in polyphenols such that it is likely that the Islander Kuna have the highest polyphenol consumption of any community in the world.

The effect of this high cocoa and polyphenol diet wasn't just reduced deaths from cardiovascular disease, but also reduced deaths from cancer and diabetes. The local Islanders had cancer rates of just 6% of their relatives eating a non-traditional diet; and deaths from diabetes were one quarter the rate of those who'd moved to the mainland.[80] Death rates from liver disease weren't specifically recorded in this publication, but deaths from gastrointestinal disease were. Gastrointestinal disease death rates in people over 60 with a high cocoa diet were half the rate of those on a non-traditional diet.

A reduction in death rates from those who have a diet high in cocoa or chocolate isn't just special to the Kuna. These results have been duplicated in many Western populations.[81] The more chocolate you have in your diet, the lower your risk of developing heart disease or dying from it. Chocolate reduces blood pressure, and improves blood vessel health and insulin levels.

Okay, so chocolate is good for my liver . . . but is it going to make me fat?

Chocolate affects your general metabolism in a positive way. It makes you more sensitive to insulin, makes your liver healthier and also reduces your risk of diabetes, heart disease and cancer. One of the fascinating things about foods that make you sensitive to insulin is that they don't seem to cause weight gain, even if they are high in calories. As we've discussed, this is because the relationship between calories and weight is not one-to-one. Insulin itself is a major driver of what happens to your weight.

Knowing that chocolate is an 'insulin sensitiser' I suspect that you could actually eat chocolate without gaining any weight from it.

This, of course, goes against common sense, which says that eating chocolate makes you fat. But what about the science?

There are several major research projects that have looked at this – with conflicting results. The first is the HELENA-CSS study from Spain (Healthy Lifestyle in Europe by Nutrition in Adolescence Cross-Sectional Study).[82] The data collected for this study was sourced from a detailed dietary and exercise history of nearly 1,400 Spanish teenagers, and included comprehensive body measurement data such as height, weight, BMI and waist circumference. This provided adequate detail to examine whether there was an effect on the teenagers' weight if they ate a lot of chocolate. The researchers concluded that the teenagers who ate the most chocolate were the leanest. They had lower weight, lower amounts of subcutaneous fat and smaller waists than their peers who ate less chocolate.[82]

Unfortunately for chocolate lovers, other more detailed studies have not been so reassuring. A larger American study interviewed more than 12,000 middle-aged men and women twice, 6 years apart, and recorded their dietary habits and weight.[83] It found that the more frequently participants ate chocolate the more weight they gained over the study. At the conclusion of the study, regular chocolate eaters (more than once a week) had put on 1 kg more weight that those who rarely ate chocolate.

Some studies suggest chocolate eaters don't put on any more weight than non-eaters, and other studies conclude the opposite. From the scientific data we currently have, it is impossible to be definitive regarding the relationship between chocolate consumption and weight gain. But here's something to think about. Many of the research studies examining chocolate and weight gain categorised all types of chocolate as simply 'chocolate'. Yet we know that milk chocolate contains more than 50% sugar and relatively small amounts of the healthy cocoa and associated polyphenols, making it a vastly different product than dark chocolate, which has less sugar and a high content of polyphenols. The studies that have looked at the issue of weight and dark chocolate specifically, have been much more reassuring. The majority suggest dark chocolate may actually reduce body weight and body fat.[84] If you enjoy chocolate and want to benefit from its liver and general health benefits, then dark chocolate is the go because foods that are insulin sensitisers typically don't result in weight gain – despite their associated calories.

Resveratrol

Resveratrol is a chemical found in grape skin and some other plant sources. The first mention of resveratrol dates back to 1939, when a Japanese scientist, Michio Takaoka, isolated it from the medicinal plant *Veratrum album*. The potential health promoting properties of resveratrol weren't reported until the 1980s, when it was found in grape skins and vines. As luck would have it, the first reports suggesting that red wine may have beneficial effects for heart health were also just then coming to public attention. Researchers then began to explore the therapeutic potential of resveratrol, pondering whether this may explain the potential health effects associated with red wine.

We now know resveratrol is in many fruits, including raspberries, blueberries and mulberries, and also nuts and other plants. In grapes, resveratrol is only in the skin. Grapes used for red wine production contain much more resveratrol than white wine grapes. It is reasonable to hypothesise that the theoretical health benefits of red wine over white is solely due to resveratrol, but there's not enough data yet to know. Interestingly, grapes produce resveratrol when the plant is under attack by pathogens such as fungi or bacteria, and it is part of a defensive mechanism to overcome the attack.

Resveratrol is anti-inflammatory, anti-oxidative and has anti-tumorigenic properties. For more than 10 years now, the microbiome (the community of bugs living in your gut) has been studied as the common pathway for how a lot of lifestyle and dietary choices affect health. The Research Centre for Nutrition and Food Safety in Chongqing, China explored how resveratrol might protect us from blood vessel damage (present in more than 80% of people over 30) by performing a series of experiments in mice to see whether resveratrol altered the gut bacteria in a way that could protect from heart disease.[85] They reported that resveratrol increased populations of health promoting bacteria and reduced bad bacteria. As a result of consuming more resveratrol, participants had lower concentrations of a chemical called trimethylamine in their blood. Lower trimethylamine meant less blood vessel damage (known as atherosclerosis, which is fatty plaques in the walls of blood vessels) and better heart health.

Add resveratrol to diet → microbiome pushes trimethylamine down → less atherosclerosis on blood vessel walls → better heart health

At present, the data on resveratrol and liver disease is generally positive. Resveratrol has been used primarily to reduce liver fat and damage, and in almost all of these studies, has been shown to have positive effects. Currently, however, the data we have is almost exclusively from research using animals, and the human data is quite preliminary.

However, there are 2 good studies. One suggests that resveratrol supplementation reduces liver fat and liver damage,[86] while the other suggests it has no effect.[87] My own personal interpretation of studies that explore whether supplements are beneficial for liver health and by implication broader health, is that they aren't. As humans we have not evolved to take resveratrol supplements in our diet. We have evolved to have berry skin that is high is resveratrol (and numerous other individual chemicals) in our diet. We don't need to complicate things looking for the health benefits from individual chemicals. Nature packaged things quite nicely for us in grapes, fruits, vegetables and other natural foods.

Foods high in resveratrol

1 Red wine
2 Red grapes
3 Peanuts
4 Pistachios
5 White wine
6 Blueberries
7 Cranberries
8 Bilberry
9 Dark chocolate
10 Other grapes

When to eat, or when not to eat

Our current culture dictates that 3 healthy meals a day offers the essential foundation to achieve good general health and longevity. Breakfast, specifically, has been anointed with special significance; according to the trope, breakfast provides us with the essential sustenance on which we can go forth and achieve the day's best. It fuels us for the morning and kills the hunger pangs that would otherwise intrude into our day. So it seems reasonable to assume that our current 3 meals a day culture has been something that has developed through evolution and has been part of human existence for millennia. This assumption however is incorrect.

The ancient Romans were obsessed with digestion and the gut and ate just one main meal a day. They believed this was healthier and aided digestion. Eating more than one meal a day was considered a form of gluttony. In the Middle Ages, only 2 meals were eaten per day. One in the middle of the day and the evening meal. Breakfast, as a word, only appeared in written English in the 15th century and literally meant to break the fast from the night before.

Do we need breakfast? During the fast between dinner and breakfast the following morning, the body maintains blood sugar levels by breaking down glycogen stored in the liver to replenish blood sugar levels. Glycogen stores in the liver are capable of maintaining blood sugar for more than 24 hours – even when fasting completely. Therefore, there is no physiological need for 3 meals every day.

Some people suggest that eating regularly and having breakfast offers protection against obesity, but this has largely been discredited in randomised controlled trials.[88] The societal pressure to consume breakfast is likely, in part, promoted by the breakfast food industry that has an obvious conflict of interest. The dogma of having 3 meals a day is actually a modern invention for which there is no evolutionary explanation and no physiological need.

The scientific evidence we do have also suggests that there is no difference to our health whether our primary meal of the day is in the morning or the evening. One small study that explored this issue was published by a Dutch research group. They enrolled 23 obese, insulin-resistant men and randomised them to a large breakfast or a large evening meal. At the end of the 4 weeks, measures of liver fat and insulin resistance were found to be equal in both groups.[89]

Eating late or snacking after your evening meal however appear to be metabolically detrimental. A large Japanese study has explored this specific area. The study from Kyushu University interviewed 2,254 individuals without fatty liver disease about a variety of eating behaviours and followed them. During the follow-up period, 52 people developed fatty liver. Eating late in the evening was associated with a 250% increased risk of developing liver disease.[90] Another Japanese study, which involved non-obese people with fatty liver, explored potential risk factors. They also found that eating within 2 hours of going to bed was associated with the development of liver disease. Night-time eating is also strongly associated with obesity and links the high rate of fatty liver disease and other metabolic complications in shift workers.

The hypothesis linking evening meals or snacks and fatty liver is centred around insulin. After each meal or snack, insulin is released into the blood to allow glucose entry into the cells.

However, if insulin levels are chronically elevated (and the cells are insulin-resistant) then excess visceral fat accumulates and fatty liver develops. With sufficient time between meals, insulin levels drop. These periods of low levels of insulin are necessary for the reversal of high insulin levels. The prolonged fast between the evening meal and eating the next day is essential to allow the necessary ebb and flow of elevated insulin to reverse.

This has very real ramifications for the best way to look after yourself: snacking is bad, fasting is good. As well as letting your insulin levels subside, I also want to mention here the fact that certain members of the microbiome flourish when there's no food in the system. It can be counter-intuitive, but a break from eating for a matter of hours can help improve diversity of the microbiome, and improve your overall health.[91]

Further data that helps consolidate the case against snacking has presented in a Dutch project led by Dr Karin Koopman.[92] Dr Koopman enrolled 36 healthy men, and for 6 weeks she put them on a high-calorie diet. The diet provided the men with 40% more calories than they needed. The men either had these calories provided during their 3 main meals or had the excess calories supplied between meals as snacks. Before the discussion that we have been through it may have been reasonable to conclude that the timing should make no difference. Conventional wisdom (which we now recognise to be incorrect) is that the problem is calorie excess, not when you eat. However, we now know that meal frequency is really important. Dr Koopman found that increasing meal frequency increased liver fat by nearly 50%, whereas no increase was seen in those men who consumed more calories during their regular 3 meals.

Fasting – fashion or fact?

Fasting or intermittent fasting has become an increasingly common topic of dinner party conversation over the last decade.

The widespread awareness of the much-touted 5/2 diet has made fasting a part of the modern health lexicon. Fasting, of course, is not a modern phenomenon. Humans have evolved to fast due to intermittent and unreliable food supplies. It is now generally accepted in the medical literature that fasting results in a number of advantageous metabolic consequences above and beyond its potential effect on weight loss. It is associated with increased lifespan, enhanced insulin sensitivity and improvements in cardiovascular risk profiles.

When people are eating 2 or 3 meals a day, the body utilises blood glucose as fuel. During periods between meals or overnight when people are fasting, glycogen in the liver is broken down and released into the blood as glucose. When you fast, the liver's supply of stored glycogen is consumed somewhere between 12 to 36 hours after the last time you ate. This timeframe depends on the liver's level of stored glycogen and your activity during this time. When liver glycogen stores are depleted, the body starts to break down stored fat to use as fuel. This is the scientific principle behind the premise that intermittent fasting may be advantageous for people to lose fat.

In some circles, fasting has become very sexy as the newly discovered key to weight loss and good health. However, it may not be all that we have hoped for. Studies that have compared weight loss between standard low-calorie diets and intermittent fasting show that neither is superior.[93] There are currently very few studies that have explored any liver health benefits from intermittent fasting.[94]

Make Mediterranean your mainstay

The liver is an amazingly complex and resilient organ. It has evolved over millions of years to process and digest thousands of different chemicals in our diets without any undue consequences. However, over more recent years, our diets have changed. The consumption of processed foods containing large amounts of sugar, particularly fructose, has challenged and overwhelmed metabolic pathways in the liver resulting in fat accumulation. To maintain liver health, limit processed foods to just occasionally and move towards the typical Mediterranean diet, with olive oil becoming a daily component of your eating.

Chapter 6

Coffee – a true food of the gods

Coffee is great for liver health. So good in fact that I'm devoting an entire chapter to sharing the existing science and the logic of why, if you don't already drink it, you should give it a shot.

Worldwide, it is estimated that 1.4 billion cups of coffee are consumed every day.[95] That's more than 500 billion cups annually. Per capita coffee consumption is led by the Scandinavian countries, with the Finnish consuming 9.6 kg of coffee per person annually and the Norwegians 7.2 kg.[96] So where is Australia? Actually, we are coffee-drinking minnows, coming in at 28th – consuming only 2.6 kg per capita annually.

Top 10 coffee consuming countries[97]

1 Finland	6 Serbia
2 Norway	7 Denmark
3 Netherlands	8 Germany
4 Slovenia	9 Belgium
5 Austria	10 Brazil

Coffee is one of the most traded commodities worldwide and worth around US$20 billion a year.

The beginning of coffee

Coffee drinking originated in current day Ethiopia. In just one of many legends, the discovery of coffee is ascribed to a 9th century Ethiopian goat herder named Kaldi. Kaldi noticed his goats become especially active after eating berries from a certain tree. After observing the energising effects of the berries, Kaldi chewed the fruit himself and felt exhilarated. He told the abbot of the local monastery who tried drinking the berries. The abbot similarly felt roused and reported improved concentration in the long hours of evening prayer. Word got around, initially among the monks in the monastery, and then beyond.

The Arabs were the first to cultivate, trade and develop a culture around coffee. Soon coffee houses opened in the Middle East and, not unlike the cafés of today, were places of conversation, dining and, perhaps most importantly, gossip. With thousands of pilgrims from all over the world visiting Mecca each year, news of the 'Wine of Araby', as coffee was often called, began to spread beyond the Arabian Peninsula. By the 17th century, coffee had made its way to Europe. There were, however, opponents – those who called coffee 'the bitter invention of Satan' – and it was condemned by many local clergy. The controversy and concern surrounding coffee became so great that the pope was asked to intervene. Pope Clement VIII tasted coffee before making a decision. He found it so satisfying that he gave it formal papal approval.

Coffee trees

Coffee plants belong to the Rubiaceae family. These evergreen trees grow up to 5 m tall and have dark green, glossy leaves, 10 cm long and about 5 cm wide. A coffee tree can survive for up to 70 years, with the first flowers typically appearing during the third year, and profitable production starting once the plant is 5 or 6 years old. Coffee berries are picked and dried to yield the seeds (or beans) inside.

Although there are approximately 60 different species of the coffee tree, just two dominate world trade: coffea arabica, which represents 75% of production; and coffea canephora, or robusta – the hardier form. The arabica is the most highly regarded and is native to the south-western highlands of Ethiopia, parts of Sudan, and northern Kenya. Coffea canephora is native to central and western sub-Saharan Africa.

The plant, caffeine and smart bees

Caffeine is just one compound in coffee, but it is the chemical directly associated with the mental stimulation you get from the drink. Why does caffeine exist? Historically, biologists thought the naturally occurring, bitter-tasting compound's main purpose was to deter herbivores from eating the coffee tree. But that didn't fully explain why caffeine has such a significant stimulatory impact.

Margaret Couvillon, from the University of Sussex in the UK, knew caffeine didn't just exist in the berry of the coffee tree, but also in some flowers. She hypothesised that the caffeine these flowers synthesised may well reflect some mutually beneficial relationship between the flowers and bees. Recent studies suggest that caffeine in flower pollen improves bees' memory so they can return to a specific plant to pollinate it next season.

In a unique experiment, Margaret Couvillion spent several days training individual bees to forage at one of 2 feeders. One of the feeders contained just sugar and water; the other, sugar, water and caffeine. Margaret demonstrated that caffeine markedly changed the bees' behaviour. The bees increased their foraging frequency and their probability and frequency of returning to the caffeine-laced sugar solution.[98] It seems that caffeine in flowers offers those plants a survival advantage.

Coffee processing

Traditionally, coffee was handpicked. Now most coffee is machine harvested, with the whole tree stripped of berries of varying ripeness. Once harvested, the flesh of the berry is removed, and the seeds fermented to get rid of the slimy layer around the seed. Then the seeds are washed and dried.

In Africa, coffee is air-dried using drying tables, but in humid climates the coffee is put into large drying cylinders. Roasting then brings the beans to 200°C, caramelising them to break down the starch and change the sugar and oil content, bringing dramatic aroma and flavour to the beans.

The caffeine in your cup

The compound that induces most of the pleasant psychological and physiological effects from a cup of coffee is caffeine. Caffeine makes up just 1–2% of the weight of the bean. It's interesting to note that by the time the liquid gets to your cup, the caffeine level can be highly variable – even if prepared by the same person, using the same equipment, day after day. Typically, an average cup of coffee contains between 50–100 mg of caffeine compared to a cup of tea, which has about half this, at 25–50 mg.

The average levels of caffeine in a standard drink

Instant coffee	60–80 mg
Latte	100–200 mg
Espresso	100 mg
Energy drinks	80 mg
Cola	50 mg
Black tea	25–100 mg
Green tea	30–50 mg
Milk chocolate	20 mg
Decaf coffee	10 mg
Iced tea	10–50 mg

Coffee also contains proteins, amino acids, carbohydrates and fibre, fats, minerals, acids and numerous polyphenols – and the levels of all of these vary depending on the method of coffee preparation. For example, cafestol and kahweol are chemicals that naturally raise cholesterol levels. These chemicals are released from roasted and ground coffee beans when hot water is in prolonged contact with the beans, but are largely removed by the paper filter used when making filtered coffee.[99]

Although the chemical composition of differently prepared coffees varies (filtered vs. non-filtered etc.), my interpretation of the literature is that there is no particular preparation that should be advocated over another. Drinkers of cafe latte, macchiato and espresso should feel equally reassured.

Coffee and the liver

Once in your body, all the numerous chemicals of coffee are broken down by the gut and liver and then excreted in the urine or bile. There is absolutely no evidence that coffee causes any sort of harm to the liver. There is, however, compelling evidence that coffee aids liver health. In the 1970s, there were several research papers that linked coffee drinking with gut cancers. This data has since been disproven, however the association between coffee and disease has given coffee a bad reputation that still lingers in some quarters.

Evidence that coffee may have liver health benefits was initially identified during studies in the 1980s and early 90s.[100,101] The first of these was undertaken by 4 Norwegian scientists and published in 1986, known as the Tromsø Heart Study (Tromsø being a region of Norway). It had previously been recognised that elevated levels of a particular liver function test, gamma-glutamyl transferase (GGT), was a marker for an increased risk of heart disease (refer back to Chapter 2 for more on liver tests). At the time, the explanation for the association between a liver test and heart disease was unknown. We now know that fatty liver disease is the link. Insulin resistance and metabolic syndrome is the common pathway leading to fatty liver disease (and increased GGT levels) and also heart disease.

The Norwegians set about examining which lifestyle factors were associated with an elevated GGT so they could identify what was causing heart disease. They surveyed and examined more than 3,000 healthy Tromsø residents, noting their age, gender, and weight, as well as lifestyle choices around alcohol, diet, cigarettes, exercise, bread, coffee and many other factors. To the surprise of the researchers, the more coffee participants drank, the lower their levels of GGT – and by implication, the better their liver health.

Let's divide the people with healthy livers into 2 groups. One group have healthy livers and don't drink coffee, the other group have healthy livers and do drink coffee. All have normal liver function tests. What was recognised by the Tromsø study, and in numerous subsequent studies, is that coffee drinkers have lower – and by this I mean better – liver function test results compared with non-drinkers. This single observation is both surprising and interesting. It means that coffee is having an effect on the liver – and is reducing liver fat, inflammation and damage! The questions that flow from this initial observation include, 'If you have a healthy liver and coffee improves your liver tests further, is that of any benefit to your health? If coffee benefits the healthy liver, does it also benefit people who already have liver disease? Can coffee protect you from liver disease? How does coffee impact your other organs?'

ALT (alanine aminotransferase) is another marker of liver inflammation, which is tested during a liver function test as we discussed in Chapter 2. Studies from Italy, Japan, and the United States have all demonstrated an inverse relationship between coffee consumption and ALT levels in the blood. Thanks to a 1993 study that involved more than 2,000 healthy Italians, we now know that the more coffee you drink, the lower your inflammation levels and the less damage there is in your liver. Those who drank 3 or more cups of coffee a day had ALT readings 10% lower than the non-coffee drinkers.[102] This reduction in ALT, although small, is important. As we discussed in Chapter 2, the lower your ALT the lower your risk of premature death.

This association between coffee and improvements in liver tests was replicated in an even larger population and published in 2014. Qian Xiao and colleagues from the National Cancer Institute, Bethesda, Maryland analysed the coffee drinking habits of more than 27,000 Americans and the relationship with their liver function tests.[103] The more coffee participants drank, the better their liver tests. Importantly, Qian Xiao performed the same analysis on people who drank decaffeinated coffee and got the same results. It appears that it is not the caffeine in coffee exerting the beneficial effects on liver health, but the other chemicals.

Following these early, simple observational studies surrounding coffee and liver enzymes, more specific trials have been performed examining whether there was any relationship between coffee consumption and liver function tests in people who have liver disease. One of these studies involved the analysis of data from nearly 6,000 Americans collected as part of the third National Health and Nutrition Examination Survey (NHANES). This study specifically examined the liver function tests of people who had risk factors for liver disease, comparing coffee drinkers with non-coffee drinkers. Participants included people who drank excessive alcohol, had hepatitis B or C, or had strong risk factors for fatty liver disease. The researchers found those with risk factors for liver disease who drank coffee were more likely to have normal liver function tests than the non-coffee drinkers. They also reported a relationship between how much coffee people drank and the protective effect. The more coffee people drank, the more likely their liver tests were to be normal. This observation is very important as it suggests there is dose response relationship between coffee and liver health.

Coffee and fatty liver disease

In research, causality can be hard to pin down. As they say, 'correlation does not prove causation'. It may be that all coffee drinkers are lean, and it is just being lean that protects people from fatty liver, with the coffee an innocent bystander. It may be that coffee drinkers exercise more, eat less or are more health literate and informed. To try and firm up the evidence for causation, a smart statistical method termed multivariable analysis helps differentiate variables that cause fatty liver disease from mere associations.

Numerous studies that use multivariable analysis have shown that while you can, of course, still develop fatty liver disease if you are a coffee drinker – it's less likely.[104,105,106] If there was a drug made by a pharmaceutical company that had this effect it would be a multi-billion-dollar product. The fact that there is something readily available, cheap, without side effects and which tastes good is remarkable.

There is no medicine out there that your doctor can prescribe that benefits your liver like a cup of coffee.

Coffee and cirrhosis

As I have described previously, cirrhosis is the medical term that defines marked scarring and permanent damage to the liver. Cirrhosis can be due to excessive alcohol intake, hepatitis B or C, fatty liver disease, immunological disease or rare genetic disorders. Several studies have examined whether coffee has any role in protecting individuals from developing cirrhosis. The majority of these studies indicate that coffee is protective, with the more you drink, the less likely your liver is to become significantly scarred and damaged.[107]

The first of these studies compared lifetime coffee non-drinkers to coffee drinkers. In these studies, the risk of cirrhosis was much lower in coffee drinkers and a relationship was demonstrated between how much coffee people drank and the reduction in their cirrhosis risk. The cirrhosis risk fell by 50%, 80% and 85% in those ingesting 1, 2, or 4 or more cups of coffee daily compared with non-coffee drinkers. Amazingly, just 2 cups of coffee a day reduced the risk of developing cirrhosis by 80%. Even after adjusting for lifestyle variables such as weight, excessive alcohol and diabetes, coffee is associated with protection against the development of cirrhosis. The more you consume, the greater the protection.[108,109]

Coffee and liver cancer

Primary liver cancer is the medical term for cancer that starts in the liver. This contrasts with secondary liver cancer – which is cancer that has spread to the liver from another site. The most common form of primary liver cancer is called hepatocellular carcinoma, or hepatoma. Most primary liver cancer occurs in people who already have an underlying liver problem. Hepatoma is increasing in frequency in many Western countries, in part, due to increasing rates of fatty liver. Worldwide, hepatoma results in approximately 700,000 deaths annually. It is the second most common cause of cancer-related death in men worldwide,[110] second only to lung cancer, and the sixth most common cause of cancer-related deaths in women.

There is now good scientific evidence that coffee reduces the risk of developing hepatoma. Population studies from Japan, Europe and Hong Kong[111-113] all uniformly report that regular coffee drinkers are relatively protected from the development of hepatoma compared to non-coffee drinkers. As with protection from cirrhosis, there is also a relationship between the amount of coffee consumed and the strength of the reduction in liver cancer risk. Some studies indicate that as little as 1–3 cups of coffee a week reduces the risk of liver cancer by approximately 50%.[112] People who drink more coffee – 5 cups daily – have their liver cancer risk reduced by up to 75%. There is currently no prescribed medication that can reduce liver cancer risk by this magnitude.

Coffee and death rates from liver disease

In medical literature, death is the ultimate end point. Yes, common sense, I know, but if you are measuring the efficacy of a new medication, the drug needs to reduce the risk of dying. For example, with medication for blood pressure, it's one thing to say the medication reduces blood pressure, or even reduces the risk of blood pressure-induced kidney damage or blood pressure-induced heart disease – but if it does these things without increasing your life expectancy, then, who cares?

In most of our discussion so far, I have presented information demonstrating coffee reduces the amount of fat in your liver, reduces liver scarring, reduces your risk of developing cirrhosis and even reduces your risk of developing liver cancer – but does it reduce your risk of dying from liver disease? If you have liver disease, this is what you want to know! Well, the evidence suggests that yes, coffee reduces your risk of dying from liver disease.

Medical research is hard work and incredibly slow. One high-quality project published in a respectable journal may be the result of several years' work by a team of health specialists.

In 2014, Dr George Boon-Bee Goh from Singapore General Hospital and colleagues from the University of Pittsburgh Cancer Institute published an article examining whether coffee intake affected the risk of dying from liver disease.[114] George and colleagues had an amazing set of data that included information on more than 63,000 middle-aged and older Chinese-Singaporeans.

The researchers analysed data previously collected for a national diet and health study.[115] The dataset included a detailed dietary history, lifestyle factors and relevant medical history for each participant. The researchers followed this cohort of people for 14 years, looked at who died, what they died from, and for any potential effect of coffee intake on the cause of death. The team was able to demonstrate that coffee drinkers were about 30% less likely to die from liver disease than non-coffee drinkers.

The researchers also looked at tea and green tea. 'Tea is good for us.' Isn't that the message? Well, that may be true for overall health, but not for the liver. Although black tea and green tea both contain caffeine, neither had any impact on the likelihood of dying from liver disease for the Singaporean cohort. As tea contains caffeine, these results also reinforce the notion that the beneficial liver effects of coffee are not from caffeine, but other compounds present in coffee.

In another study[116] looking at the effect of caffeine on blood pressure, one group were given coffee and the other group a pill with the equivalent dose of caffeine. Instinctively, you might expect both groups to experience a similar impact on their blood pressure; after all, both groups received the same amount of caffeine. But that's not what happened. Blood pressure increased by an average of 1mmHg for the coffee drinkers, but 3mmHg for those taking the caffeine pills. This effect is small, of course, but is important in illustrating that the effects of coffee and caffeine can be quite different. And again, it appears the liver benefits are from coffee, not caffeine.

Coffee and the liver – boiling it down

Controversy regarding the health benefits or hazards of coffee still exists in some circles, but the overwhelming evidence from experimental and population-based studies is that coffee has significant benefits. Coffee reduces liver fat (a crucial initial step in liver injury from all causes), reduces progression of liver scarring, reduces liver cancer risk and reduces your risk of dying from liver disease.

A liver panacea? Not quite, but probably the closest thing we currently have to one.

One of the concerns in the scientific community – which I mentioned during the discussion on fatty liver – is that a lot of the data on coffee comes from association studies. These studies demonstrate an association, but don't prove causation. Increasingly though, mechanistic studies demonstrating the beneficial physiological effects of coffee are being performed, and the results are promising.

As the association studies describing the positive liver health benefits of coffee have matured, some mechanistic studies have been undertaken. One such project examined caffeic acid, one of the hundreds of compounds in a cup of coffee. Caffeic acid was shown to suppress the growth of the hepatitis C virus.[117] More recently, studies have demonstrated that coffee protects the liver from fructose-induced fatty liver damage and insulin resistance.[118] This important finding may help explain how coffee protects individuals from many of the diseases related to poor diet and insulin resistance.

New data has demonstrated that chlorogenic acid, another compound in coffee, induces changes in gut bacterial populations.[119] As we have discussed, gut bacteria may be one of the common pathways by which obesity, insulin resistance and its complications create disease. So, food, exercise and lifestyle most likely influence health via changes in the microbiome – which means it's actually the microbiome that causes leaky gut and exposes the liver (and other body systems) to toxic chemicals when the gut flora is unhealthy.

The data we have regarding coffee and liver health is largely based on association studies. Association by itself does not prove causation. However, the magnitude and reproducibility of the findings regarding coffee and liver health is compelling. The next steps are interventional studies, prospective randomised trials, where people with liver disease are given coffee or a placebo and liver function and liver fat compared between the 2 groups. At present these trials have not been performed, but are eagerly awaited.

Coffee and brown fat

There are 2 types of fat present in humans. The majority of our fat tissue is white fat, but we also carry brown fat. Brown fat makes up a large percentage of total body fat in newborns, but gradually falls as a percentage of total body fat as we age. In adults, brown fat is carried in tissues around the neck, and its main function is to help control body temperature. Brown fat contains a much higher concentration of mitochondria than white fat, and it is the mitochondria that give brown fat its colour. Mitochondria are the energy producing parts of our cells. In brown fat they turn glucose and fat into energy, thereby increasing body temperature and also burning calories to control body weight.

Interestingly, a recent report revealed that caffeine increases the activity of brown fat. The researchers from the University of Nottingham in the UK randomised a small number of participants to drink either a glass of water or a cup of instant coffee. Then they measured brown fat activity by assessing the temperature of the skin around the neck. Skin temperature increased in those drinking coffee, whereas no effect was seen in those drinking water.[120] The effect was small and not enough that coffee could be advocated as a weight loss strategy via this mechanism but is another potential pathway by which coffee exerts its positive metabolic effects.

Coffee and the other organs

Well, I may have hopefully convinced you that coffee is good for your liver, but it is essential to also look at coffee's impact on other organs as well. It's less than optimal, obviously, if coffee stops you dying of liver disease but causes you to die of some other health problem. In the next section, I discuss the data that examines the impact of coffee on the other major organs and common diseases.

Coffee and heart health

As coffee is consumed by such a large proportion of the population, and heart disease is very common, even potentially small health benefits or risks associated with drinking coffee may have important public health implications. And as a result, the effects of coffee on the cardiovascular system have been closely examined, with the weight of evidence indicating coffee is beneficial for your heart. Good news.

High blood pressure (hypertension) is a major risk factor for heart disease and stroke. My guess is that if you asked 100 people whether coffee increases blood pressure, the majority would say yes. But that majority would be wrong. One recent large analysis that pooled the results of 15 studies examining coffee intake and blood pressure, found no relationship between long-term coffee consumption and blood pressure.[121] Coffee consumption has been associated with minor transient increases in blood pressure, but only in people who aren't regular coffee drinkers. In regular drinkers, coffee has no effect on blood pressure. There is even data suggesting coffee may slightly lower your blood pressure if you are a non-smoker.[122]

Diabetes is another major risk factor for heart disease. Most adult-onset diabetes is due to insulin resistance – which we talked about in Chapter 2. Coffee reduces insulin resistance, making the body more sensitive to the beneficial effects of this hormone. Coffee drinkers are relatively protected from developing diabetes compared to non-coffee drinkers. The more coffee you drink, the more you are protected. Heavy drinkers of coffee (more than 6 cups a day) are more protected than moderate drinkers (2–4 cups a day), who are more protected than people who only drink one cup a day.[123]

> Insulin is the most important hormone in the regulation of blood sugar; therefore, as the body becomes resistant to the effects of insulin, blood sugar levels rise, ultimately leading to diabetes.

Cholesterol is another major risk factor for heart disease. Here however, the news is not so good for coffee. As I mentioned earlier, coffee contains 2 cholesterol increasing compounds; cafestol and kahweol. The concentrations of these compounds are higher in boiled coffee as the chemicals are drawn from the coffee by prolonged contact with hot water. This contrasts with filtered coffee, where the contact time with hot water is shorter and the compounds are removed by the paper filter. If you have high cholesterol and your doctor feels you are at risk of heart disease, ask your doctor whether coffee is fine to continue or best avoided. Interestingly, tea has the reverse effect on cholesterol, lowering 'bad' LDL cholesterol and elevating 'good' HDL cholesterol.[124]

Coffee and death from heart disease

So, some good and some potentially not-so-good effects for the heart if you are a coffee drinker. Coffee reduces your risk of diabetes, has no real effect on your blood pressure, but may increase your cholesterol. If you want to look at the big picture, the most important question is whether coffee alters your risk of dying from heart disease – especially given that heart disease kills one in 4 people in the Western world. If I'm a coffee drinker, does coffee make me more likely or less likely to die of heart disease?

The authors of the HAPIEE (which stands for Health, Alcohol and Psychological Factors In Eastern Europe) study explored the potential of coffee to protect people from dying of heart disease. Researchers collected dietary data, including coffee consumption, on more than 28,000 Eastern Europeans.[125] The research revealed that the more coffee you drank, the lower your risk of dying from heart disease. Importantly, the size of the protective effect was quite marked. During the study, men who drank 1–2 cups of coffee a day had a 10% lower risk of cardiovascular death, while women had a 32% lower risk. Men who drank 3–4 cups a day reduced their risk by almost 30%. This protective association between coffee intake and cardiovascular health isn't only true for the inhabitants of Eastern Europe. The same protective association has been demonstrated for coffee drinkers in numerous other populations.[126]

Coffee and longevity

In May 2012, scientists from Washington DC published an intriguing article in the most prestigious medical journal in the world, *The New England Journal of Medicine*.[127] The study explored a database of diet and lifestyle factors of 400,000 individuals that began in 1995, continuing for the next 13 years. Overall, the database had more than five million person-years of follow up. The title of the article was 'Association of coffee drinking with total and cause-specific mortality'. The article is available on the internet and is a really interesting read. So, what did the researchers find? Coffee drinking is associated with a reduced risk of death from heart disease, respiratory disease, stroke, injuries and accidents, diabetes and infections, and is an insulin sensitiser. Coffee reduces insulin levels, and, as we discussed in the first chapter, high levels of insulin drives many of the common diseases of the Western world. Coffee makes you live longer and healthier. It offers protection from not just liver disease, but many of the leading causes of death worldwide.

Adverse effects of coffee

Every drug that exerts an effect has the potential to cause side effects. Coffee is no exception. The amazing thing about coffee, however, is that the side effect profile is generally benign, and most people can tolerate a cup or 2 a day quite well. However, with higher doses, some people complain of anxiety or disrupted sleep. High coffee intake has also been associated with an increased risk of osteoporosis in women.[128] The reason for this is that coffee causes an increased loss of calcium in the urine. However, adding a dash of milk to your cup offsets the calcium loss in the urine. If you are a heavy (more than 5 cups a day) coffee drinker, I suggest you consciously boost your dietary intake of calcium-rich foods such as full-fat yoghurt.

The risks of caffeine-based energy drinks

The last decade or two has seen the introduction of a new food: the 'energy drink'. As far as I can recall, when I was a child this group of products didn't exist. But now energy drinks are well and truly embedded in the mainstream. According to Euromonitor, global sales of energy drinks have leapt from A$4 billion in 1999 to A$30 billion in 2013. There are of course, multiple different recipes for these drinks, but most contain caffeine and sugar, and some contain guarana as well, which also contains caffeine. Most energy drinks contain no more caffeine than a typical cup of coffee, however the sugary taste of these drinks makes them attractive to children and an emerging problem is teenagers experiencing dangerous side effects from drinking too much too quickly.

Very high doses of caffeine can result in a variety of symptoms including irritability, stomach upset, palpitations and insomnia. In 2011 in the United States, it was estimated that energy drinks resulted in 20,000 attendances to the emergency department.[129] Typically, people don't develop side effects from caffeine unless greater than 400 mg (the equivalent of 4–8 cups of coffee) is consumed, which translates to drinking 4 or more energy drinks in a very short time-span.

In one Australian study, of people ringing the poisons information centre with symptoms of caffeine excess from energy drinks, nearly 50% required hospitalisation and 8% had life-threatening symptoms, including serious cardiac complications, seizures, hallucinations and heart damage.[130] Deaths from these drinks have also been reported.[131] Government-led regulation of these drinks now seems timely. Enforcing sales restrictions to children and encouraging industry regulation to market these products responsibly are also very appropriate initial measures.

A case history – caffeine overdose

'The decedent was a 39-year-old white man who had been employed as a telecommunications worker. The decedent was physically active and participated in a demanding daily fitness regime, which included the preparation and consumption of self-formulated "energy drinks". His employer had recently received several complaints about the decedent, predominately related to his aggressive behaviour. As a result, the decedent was terminated from his position. Approximately 2 hours after his termination, the decedent was found lifeless at the front door of his residence by a friend. Emergency medical services were called, but no vital signs were identified. No suicide note or evidence of suicidal ideation was found.'

The autopsy examination revealed the deceased had consumed 10–12 g of caffeine, the equivalent of 100–120 energy drinks. The coroner concluded that the caffeine had caused the man's heart to stop resulting in his death. The medical literature includes more than 40 reports of death from caffeine overdose. The minimum dose reported to result in a death is 5 g – about 100 cups of coffee or 50 energy drinks.[132]

Coffee, caffeine and the Olympics

As we all know, caffeine is a stimulant; that's one of the reasons we drink coffee. It's also the reason why caffeine is added to many soft drinks, almost all energy drinks and is popular with the professional sporting community. While caffeine is legally acceptable for athletes now, this was not always the case. In years gone by, it was okay for athletes to drink coffee and compete, but not for them to take caffeine supplements. The International Olympics Committee (IOC) set a level of caffeine in the urine that was acceptable, based on the upper limit of normal for people drinking coffee. By implication, any level above this was considered to be the result of doping with caffeine supplements and deemed as cheating.

In 1988, Alex Watson was a pentathlete for Australia at the Seoul Olympics. After a daylong series of fencing bouts Watson was randomly selected for a urine test. The test came back positive for caffeine at a concentration of 14 mcgs per ml – the IOC upper allowable limit was 12 mcgs per ml. The following day the IOC Board banned Watson from further participation at the Seoul Olympics, making him the first member of the Australian Olympic team to be disqualified at an Olympic games for a drug-related offence. What followed was a media storm. Alex Watson organised a media conference protesting his innocence and a number of medical experts came forward supporting his assertion that the coffee he had drunk was enough to cause the high urine concentration without having taken a caffeine supplement.

Professor Birkett, a professor of pharmacology from Flinders University was then employed by the TV station Channel Ten to see whether the concentration of caffeine in Alex Watson's urine could have just come from drinking coffee and Coca-Cola. In an experiment, Professor Birkett revealed identical urine concentrations of caffeine as the original test had shown when Alex drank 10 cups of coffee and 2 cans of Coca-Cola. Eventually, Alex Watson cleared his name and went on to compete in the 1992 Barcelona Olympics.

Is coffee/caffeine dehydrating (does it make you wee more)?

Of some concern to my sporting science colleagues, is the potential disadvantage caffeine could have if it makes you urinate excessively. There have been at least 15 different studies that looked at the potential diuretic (urine producing) effect of coffee. And here's the deal: if you are having 2 or less cups of coffee a day, you lose no more fluid than someone having the equivalent amount of fluid as water. If you have between 2 and 6 cups of coffee daily, then the data on coffee's diuretic effect is at best equivocal.[133]

So, it seems that most of the diuretic effect we associate with coffee is due to the water content of the coffee, rather than any specific effect of coffee on the kidneys. If you drink more, you'll urinate more!

Just when you thought you knew all there was to know about coffee – the science of the coffee ring

I have no doubt you've seen it on your newspaper; the particular ring-like stain left after a coffee spill. The shape of the stain; light in the middle and dark around the edges is specifically referred to in the scientific community as the 'coffee ring effect'.

According to Robert Deegan from the University of Chicago, writing in the prestigious science journal *Nature*, the pattern of coffee flow on a surface is due to capillary flow induced by variable evaporation rates across the spill.[134] Liquid evaporating from the edge of the stain is replenished by liquid from the interior. The resulting edgeward flow carries almost all the dissolved coffee to the edge of the stain. Although these observations may seem inane, they have proved essential in the design of equipment from the ink-jet printer to diagnostic sensors for blood-based analysis.

And so?

Coffee is great. It really is a wonder drug when it comes to liver health. If your liver is already good, coffee makes it better. If your liver is not so flash, coffee improves it. And if your liver is sick, coffee reduces your risk of liver cancer and death from liver failure. Apart from its beneficial effects on the liver, coffee has protective effects against lung disease, heart disease, stroke, diabetes and infections.[127] Coffee drinkers live longer. If you enjoy coffee, keep drinking it. If you avoid it because of perceived ill effects, you might want to reconsider.

Chapter 7

Alcohol – friend or foe?

Socially, when I say I'm a liver specialist, there is often some comment about alcohol. People imagine me to be a puritanical teetotaller. But I am actually quite the opposite. I'm quite fun (once you get to know me) and I enjoy a drink. I don't enjoy all types of alcohol. Spirits remind me of bad hangovers as a younger man, beer makes me feel bloated, but wine? Wine, I thoroughly enjoy.

The fact that people are surprised that a liver specialist enjoys alcohol relates, of course, to the fact that alcohol causes liver disease and therefore people think I should know better. The truth though, is that for most individuals, alcohol can be beneficial – rather than detrimental. For decades we have heard the message that alcohol causes cirrhosis, alcohol is a drug of addiction and alcohol ruins lives and, of course, all of these things are true. But it doesn't have to be like that. When it is abused, alcohol can be as potentially devastating to people's lives as heroin. However, modest alcohol intake almost certainly does more good than harm.

The history of alcohol and humans

Alcohol has been a part of human society dating back at least 9,000 years. Chemical analysis of traces of residue from ancient Chinese pottery confirms these vessels were used for drinks of fermented grape, hawthorn fruit wine and rice beer. The Egyptians were enjoying alcohol 5,000 years ago and the Sudanese 3,500 years ago. Alcohol in our bodies is broken down by a specific enzyme in the liver called alcohol dehydrogenase (ADH). Humans, and all primates, have this enzyme.

Actually, our capacity to metabolise alcohol goes back even further. Our gut bacteria are not just involved in the breakdown of food, but appear to be a factory for the synthesis of essential chemicals and vitamins, as well as playing an integral role in the regulation of our general metabolism and immune function. Gut bacteria also produces alcohol from the fermentation of food we eat. The amount of alcohol produced by the gut bacteria is enough for it to be detectable in our blood. Our ancient ancestors needed an enzyme to break down alcohol, as alcohol production in the gut of humans, primates and all animals has been going on for millions of years.

Humans and modern primates (chimpanzees and gorillas) have a form of ADH that is 40 times more efficient at breaking down alcohol than the form seen in more primitive primate species, such as the marmoset, macaque and orangutan.[135] This suggests that the highly efficient form of ADH evolved about 10 million years ago when humans, chimpanzees and gorillas shared a common ancestor. It is hypothesised that the single amino acid mutation that occurred in the ADH enzyme to make it the more active form occurred as our ancient ancestors increasingly travelled along the forest floor and consumed more fermented fruits containing alcohol.[135]

It is a fact that alcohol has been part of primate/human evolution dating back millions of years. This means it isn't some modern chemical creation that our bodies can't handle. Indeed, the opposite is true. Natural alcohol production within our bodies continues today in modern humans and is generated 24/7 in all of us.

The ability to consume alcohol may have shaped primate evolution. The enzyme that breaks down alcohol in humans evolved 10 million years ago and offered a survival advantage for primitive apes.

The alcohol in all of us

The microorganisms in our gut convert some of our dietary carbohydrates into alcohol and carbon dioxide. The alcohol produced can be as much as 20 g a day, which is the equivalent of 2 standard alcoholic drinks,[136] although the amount produced depends very much on what we eat and the type of microorganisms we have in our gut. Most often, it's not much, but occasionally it can actually be enough to make people ill. Makes you wonder what's going on in your gut when you feel like a lie down after a big meal. One startling medical publication describes the story of a 5-year-old boy in Uganda who died after his stomach exploded because of the fermentation of a large meal of sweet potato.[137]

The gut producing enough alcohol to make a person unwell is, of course, extremely rare. The medical term for this condition is 'autobrewery syndrome'. As you can imagine, it must be tempting for savvy lawyers to attempt to use this as a defence in drink-driving cases. And of course, this has been attempted, although unsuccessfully. The amount of alcohol produced by our gut that is detectable in our blood or breath is at least 10 times lower than the drink driving level of 0.05%.[138] However, it may also go some way to explaining why small amounts of alcohol appear to be good for us.

What can potentially happen when the gut microorganisms get out of hand

After repeated episodes of apparent intoxication, a 13-year-old girl in America was diagnosed as being drunk based on high blood alcohol levels. The girl, however, denied drinking any alcohol. She was admitted to a rehabilitation facility where she was continuously monitored, had no access to alcohol, yet still displayed intoxicated behaviour and had elevated blood alcohol levels. Ultimately, doctors came to the conclusion she was producing alcohol in her own gut by fermentation.

The family noted that these episodes tended to occur after she ingested excess carbohydrates and juices. Eventually, a strong correlation was found between her elevated alcohol levels and intake of high carbohydrate meals or fructose-containing drinks. She subsequently underwent a gastroscopy where her gut flora was sampled to see which specific organism might be causing the problem. High yeast levels were treated with antibiotics and the girl's symptoms resolved.[139] The girl had a history of gut resection as a child, which had predisposed her bowel to colonisation by high levels of yeast.

Humans evolved to drink alcohol – wild fermentation

It is estimated that 90% of the population in Western countries have consumed alcohol at some stage in their adult life, 70% in the past year and 55% in the past month. These numbers are extraordinarily high – why are humans drawn to consume alcohol?

In nature, the primary source of alcohol is fermented sugars from fruit created by naturally occurring yeasts. Fruit trees use birds and animals as a mechanism for spreading the plant's seeds over a wide area. The more attractive a plant can make its fruit, the greater the survival advantage it gains. As fruit ripens, the sugar content increases and birds and mammals are drawn to it. Unripe fruit, by contrast, has unripe seeds, not ready for propagation and the fruit is often bitter and unattractive – discouraging animals from taking it before it is ripe.

Yeasts involved in fruit decay are present both inside fruit and on the external surface. As fruit starts to ripen the naturally occurring sugars are fermented by the yeast resulting in the production of alcohol. The alcohol produced inhibits the growth of bacteria and therefore slows the breakdown of the fruit, allowing more time for it to be eaten and the seeds dispersed.

Alcohol produced by the fruit smells sweet, creating a sensory stimulus for primates and other animals, and provides a significant caloric reward. There are almost twice as many calories in a gram of alcohol as in a gram of sugar, which means the calorie gain from consuming overripe fruits offered a survival advantage to our ancient ancestors.

We're not the only primates taking a tipple

In 2016, Samuel Gochman and 2 colleagues from the USA performed experiments exploring whether primates prefer alcohol containing foods over and above non-alcohol containing foods. Using 2 different types of monkey, the Slow Loris and the Aye-Aye (both great looking species, look them up on Google), researchers set up a table with cups of sugary liquid that simulated their natural diet of nectar. To some of these sugary drinks the researchers added various amounts of alcohol, from 1% to 5%, with the aim of trying to discover whether monkeys can detect alcohol, and whether they like it. The answer to both questions was yes. The monkeys preferred the alcohol-containing solutions to the sugar-only drink, and the higher-alcohol-content drinks over the low-alcohol alternatives.[140]

Scientific evidence of our primate relatives seeking out alcohol in the natural environment has been well documented. In Guinea, West Africa, long-term and recurrent ingestion of alcohol has been reported in a group of wild chimpanzees studied over nearly 20 years.[141] In this region of Guinea, the sugars in the raffia palm naturally ferments to produce alcohol, and local villagers tap the palm, causing the sap to drip into a large container they place by the tree. The tappers collect all the fermented sap in the morning and then again in the evening. For years though, the locals have known they are competing with chimpanzees for the intoxicating sap – and recently, video cameras were set up around several tapped raffia palms to explore the drinking culture of this troop of chimpanzees.

The sap contains between 3% and 7% alcohol, similar to most beer. The chimpanzees were observed breaking off a palm leaf, scrunching it up in their mouths to form a spoon-shaped tool, and then dipping the leaf into the collecting container to drink the liquid. Across the troop, drinking habits varied significantly. Occasionally, one chimpanzee would monopolise the container, while at other times the drink was shared between many. Overall, about half the troupe participated (age and gender seemed irrelevant). The troop drank between 3 and 85 ml of alcohol in a session (the upper range has an alcohol content similar to a bottle of wine). Some of the chimpanzees appeared drunk after consuming the alcohol with others resting immediately after their drink. Individual chimpanzees returning repeatedly to the palm sap suggests alcohol ingestion was a conscious choice.

So, why do chimpanzees seek out alcohol? Hormesis is a biological phenomenon whereby a beneficial health impact results from low doses of an agent that is potentially toxic or lethal at higher doses. Alcohol is the perfect example of this principle. Humans have evolved to be continually exposed to small amounts of alcohol from the endogenous production in our gut flora. Primates (and by implication modern humans), have evolved to seek out alcohol because of its potential to offer a survival advantage. In this context, alcoholism is viewed as a disease of nutrient excess, much like obesity is viewed as a consequence of a nutrient excess of our modern diet.

How much alcohol is in alcoholic drinks?

Alcoholic drinks vary markedly in how much alcohol they contain. Light beers may be only 1 or 2% alcohol, whereas some spirits may be 40–50% alcohol. A standard serve of alcohol or 'standard drink' in Australia contains 10 g of alcohol, whether it be beer, wine or spirits. For example, a standard drink of beer (4.8% alcohol) is 200 ml with 10 g of alcohol; wine (11.5% alcohol) is 100 ml with 10 g of alcohol; and a high strength spirit called a nip, of 30 ml, also contains about 10 g of alcohol. Where it gets confusing is if we pour more than a standard serve into our glass and therefore consume greater than 10 g of alcohol in a drink. This is what often happens in restaurants; a glass of wine in a restaurant typically contains about 150 ml, which is one and a half standard drinks. Red wine (often about 13% alcohol content) has a higher alcohol concentration than white wine (usually about 11% alcohol), adding to the confusion. This means the glass of red wine you are served in a restaurant may contain 20 g of alcohol – which is the equivalent of 2 standard drinks.

Keep in mind, that when I talk about moderate alcohol intake, I mean up to 2 units of alcohol for women and up to 3 units for men on any given day, with a maximum of 7 units for women and 14 for men over a week.

A healthy liver can manage moderate alcohol intake

As we discussed in Chapter 1, the normal healthy liver is a chemical factory. Its job is to filter bad chemicals from the blood and manufacture good chemicals. Most of the bad chemicals the liver filters out are broken down remnants of what we've eaten. There's nothing to worry about – this is, after all, the liver's primary role. The plant-based foods we eat are made up of thousands of different compounds. All the blood from the gut (including chemicals we have eaten) drains through the liver – and the liver takes out the bad stuff, keeps the good stuff and manufactures essential chemicals.

Alcohol therefore (in moderation), is metabolised by the healthy liver without any issue. As we have discussed, even if you don't drink alcohol, your gut is making it 24/7 and your liver is therefore metabolising alcohol 24/7. Adding small quantities of alcohol to your diet is not going to bother your liver one bit.

The liver's role in breaking down alcohol

The liver can break down approximately 10 g of alcohol (one standard drink) per hour in the average individual. If you drink 2 drinks in an hour (20 g of alcohol) it will take your liver about 2 hours to break it down. Drinking more than a standard drink per hour results in the accumulation of alcohol in your blood, which leads to feeling drunk. The rate of alcohol metabolism can vary up to 3–4 times between individuals. Alcohol metabolism is higher in men than women due purely to the difference in size between the individuals. If you compare liver size – gram for gram between the sexes – then women actually have slightly faster alcohol metabolisation rates. Alcohol elimination between races is generally similar. Rates of alcohol metabolism by Caucasians and Asians are overall similar, although liver size (being, on average, smaller in Asians) may explain some slight differences. Having a meal with alcohol accelerates its metabolism compared with the fasted state. There is also variation in alcohol elimination rates according to the time of day, with the best time to have a drink at the end of the day.[142]

About the available data

Some of the studies I cite in this chapter on the potential health benefits of alcohol describe circumstantial links between health and alcohol, and have been gleaned from interviewing people who have a disease, then interviewing healthy people and looking for the differences. This means that while there is a proven link, there's no proven cause and effect. So, we need to be somewhat cautious in interpreting the potential health benefits of alcohol, and remember that all the positive outcomes are based on *moderate* consumption.

Can alcohol be good for you?

Alcoholic drinks contain numerous chemicals, not just alcohol (ethanol) and water. Wine, for example, has minerals (magnesium, calcium, potassium, copper, zinc and iron), sugars, proteins, polyphenols, glutathione, dissolved carbon dioxide and more. Medicine is a reductionist science. What I mean by reductionist is that when we see cause and effect scientists will try and distil (no apology for the pun) it down to the specific ingredient in that food or drink that causes that result. Therefore, when we get to alcoholic drinks and liver health, it is tempting to look at the list of ingredients and try and explain which of the natural chemicals in wine (or other alcoholic drinks) results in the health benefits. In medicine, the results are most often disappointing when scientists try and explore the individual components of food and look for positive health benefits. This is true of vitamins and minerals (with the possible exception of vitamin D) and other analysis on individual compounds such as resveratrol. Generally, the individual components of food aren't associated with liver health benefits, it's more about whole foods.

Are the health benefits purely an effect of the ethanol? We know that it's not just wine that has health benefits but all the alcohol containing drinks, and we know that our gut flora makes ethanol; maybe it's just the ethanol. But really, we don't know.

Alcohol and fatty liver disease

By now you are an expert on fatty liver disease. You know it is a lifestyle disease, typically caused by eating the wrong foods, being overweight and/or doing too little exercise. These lifestyle choices elevate insulin levels and the insulin drives fat into the liver cells, starting a potential cascade of inflammation and liver damage.

In fact, moderate alcohol intake appears to make people more insulin-sensitive, and compared to non-drinkers, moderate drinkers have lower insulin levels and a lower risk of developing fatty liver disease.[146,147] The opposite is true for heavy drinkers; heavy alcohol intake of more than 3 standard drinks a day is associated with elevated insulin levels and a higher risk of developing fatty liver disease.

One Japanese study looked at 8,000 healthy people who underwent a detailed health check-up – including screening for fatty liver disease. The people in the study filled in a comprehensive health questionnaire looking at general lifestyle factors, such as level of exercise, smoking, alcohol intake, height, weight, and blood pressure. What the researchers found was that there were only 2 factors that appeared to protect individuals from fatty liver; they were regular exercise and alcohol consumption. Amazingly, of these 2 factors, alcohol offered individuals greater protection from liver damage then regular exercise did.[145] An even larger study reported data from 43,000 individuals. According to the findings, people drinking moderate amounts of alcohol had a 30–40% reduction in the risk of developing fatty liver compared with non-drinkers. This association persisted even after correcting for body weight, the strongest recognised risk factor for fatty liver.

Of course, moderate drinking doesn't totally prevent people getting fatty liver, it just reduces the likelihood.

If you've visited your local doctor and been told you have fatty liver disease, should you stop drinking all together? Well, if you drink too much then, yes. (Remember, too much is more than one or 2 standard drinks daily, 4 days a week for women, and more than 3 standard drinks a day up to 4 days a week for men.) But what if you are a moderate (i.e. only drink up to the levels I've suggested) drinker? Can alcohol ever be good for you if you have liver disease? Well, this is a really big question and the answer needs to be taken in context. Here we go.

Reassuringly, and perhaps surprisingly, the evidence is that moderate alcohol intake for people with fatty liver disease does not worsen their liver disease, and appears to improve it, at least in some studies.[143-145] As I alluded to earlier, most people with fatty liver disease don't die of their liver disease – the most common causes of death in patients with fatty liver disease are heart attack, stroke or cancer. And there is now increasing evidence that alcohol appears to protect the liver from developing fatty liver disease.

In some studies,[144,148] moderate alcohol consumption was associated with a reduced risk of the 'nasty' form of fatty liver (NASH), compared to not drinking at all. NASH is the form of fatty liver disease where there is significant inflammation in the liver. This is the form of fatty liver disease most likely to progress to cirrhosis and liver cancer.

If you already have a liver problem, is all alcohol harmful?

If you're thinking, I have fatty liver disease, and don't drink, should I start? Well, my suggestion would be that you don't start. We don't yet have enough evidence to suggest that non-drinkers with fatty liver disease start drinking. Suggesting that would be irresponsible.

But if you have fatty liver disease and drink modestly, I see no reason why you should stop – keep enjoying it. However, if you have liver disease from excessive alcohol consumption, don't drink alcohol at all. For liver disease due to causes other than fatty liver, there is no evidence that even moderate alcohol is worth the risk. The liver benefits of moderate alcohol consumption appear to be specifically for fatty liver disease and not associated with other causes of liver injury.

The French embrace

Two decades ago, an article in the prestigious medical journal *The Lancet* coined the term 'The French Paradox'. The paradox was that the French – despite a diet high in saturated fats (historically these are bad fats) – had a low incidence of death from cardiac disease. The explanation for this apparent disparity was the moderate alcohol consumption typical of the French diet – and the premise that moderate alcohol intake protected the heart. Ever since, there has been growing evidence moderate alcohol intake doesn't just protect individuals from fatty liver disease and heart disease, but also against diabetes, dementia and numerous other conditions. Although we still don't know why, alcohol has been shown to be antioxidant, anti-inflammatory, blood pressure lowering and have anticoagulant properties. All these are good.

Alcohol and your heart

Moderate alcohol intake is good for heart health. Heart disease is the most common cause of death in Western society, and moderate alcohol intake reduces your risk of cardiovascular death by about 25%;[147,149] but again, let me say it: it is essential to stress moderate, and that's a lot less than many of us have grown accustomed to.

Now back to your heart. Cardiovascular disease impacts the heart and blood vessels. If you have cardiovascular disease, it means fat is deposited in the walls of the blood vessels, gradually narrowing the channels and reducing their ability to carry blood. If fat is deposited in the wall of a blood vessel, the vessel wall can split, and then a blood clot forms on the top of the fatty deposit, which can totally block the blood vessel, and blood flow is stopped completely. A heart attack is the lay term used when this event occurs in one of the blood vessels taking blood to your heart. This results in part of the heart muscle being starved of blood and dying. This, in turn, leads to permanent heart damage or death. Blood vessel damage can cause reduced blood flow in any part of the body. When it happens in your brain, it is a stroke; but it can also occur in your kidney vessels, your gut vessels or the blood vessels in your legs. Moderate alcohol use is associated with reduced blood vessel damage from fat, reduced blood fats (triglycerides), and increased insulin sensitivity. It also thins the blood, reducing the risk of clots.

Your risk of a heart attack is proportional to the blood vessel damage from fatty cholesterol deposits. As the deposits age, calcium is deposited in the plaques – the plaques become calcified. The amount of calcium in these fatty deposits is a marker of heart attack risk. Moderate drinkers have lower levels of calcium in the cardiac blood vessels and are therefore at lower risk of heart attack, compared with non-drinkers and heavier drinkers.[150]

Alcohol and diabetes

Type 2 diabetes is a lifestyle-related disease, predominantly impacting people who are overweight and/or who do too little exercise. Type 2 diabetes makes sufferers resistant to insulin (the primary hormone involved in blood sugar control), causing increased insulin levels and elevated blood sugar levels. It is estimated that up to 4% of Australians, or one in 25, currently have diabetes.

Moderate alcohol consumption improves the body's sensitivity to insulin. This means moderate drinkers have a lower risk of developing type 2 diabetes, a finding that has been demonstrated in multiple research studies.[151-153] The magnitude of alcohol's impact in reducing diabetes risk is significant. One research project reported the pooled findings from 15 smaller studies involving 370,000 people followed for more than a decade. It concluded that people who drank moderate amounts of alcohol had a 30% lower risk of developing type 2 diabetes that non-drinkers or heavier drinkers.

This reduced risk of developing diabetes with moderate alcohol intake is true for both men and women and appears to be independent of the person's weight. The effect is also independent of the type of alcohol consumed. The benefit is observed with drinkers of wine, beer and spirits. It is important to note that heavier drinking is a risk factor for diabetes, with the risk increasing the more people drink. Heavier drinkers not only lose the protective effect of alcohol, but significantly increase their risk of developing diabetes.

For women, moderate drinking refers to no more than 7 standard drinks a week, with only 2 drinks in any given day, and at least one alcohol free day a week.

So, what does 'heavier' alcohol consumption look like? If you are drinking a bottle of wine over the course of a week, it's already too much.

Alcohol and dementia

As the average age of a society increases, the proportion of people affected by dementia is also increasing. It is so common in our society that it is likely most of us have a family member or friend affected by the disease. Dementia robs people of their personalities and independence – and there is no effective therapy to halt or reverse it. There are many different forms of dementia, with Alzheimer's disease the most common.

Dementia is a brain-altering disease, and alcohol is a drug that can affect your brain, so it's reasonable to conclude that alcohol is a risk factor for dementia. However, the opposite is actually true. Several studies have followed older people without dementia over time and compared the rate of developing the disease between moderate drinkers and non-drinkers. All the studies have come to the same conclusion – moderate alcohol intake is associated with a reduced risk of developing dementia (and Alzheimer's disease). This reduction in dementia risk appears to be between 20 and 40%. The conclusions of many of these observational studies are supported by reports that reveal that alcohol reduces damage to nerve synapses by plaques that occur in Alzheimer's disease.[154]

Alcohol and stroke

Stroke is caused by either the blocking of an artery supplying blood to part of the brain or a haemorrhage into the brain. The resulting brain injury from a lack of blood results in permanent damage. If the stroke is from a blood clot, then early treatment with clot-busting medications can limit the brain injury. Brain damage may result in a variety of symptoms, depending on which part of the brain is affected by the stroke. It may affect the speech centre, resulting in either an inability to speak or jumbled speech, or it may affect the arms and legs of the patient resulting in permanent weakness and/or stiffness of the involved limb/s.

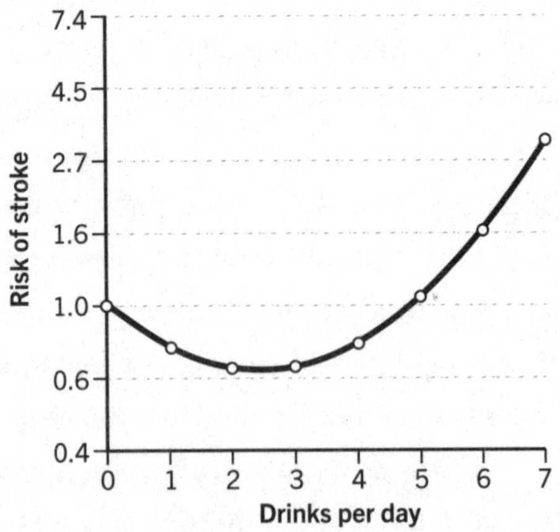

Figure 7.1 The 'J' shaped relationship between alcohol intake and risk of stroke.

Stroke is a major cause of death and disability in all Western counties. Many studies have explored whether there is a relationship between alcohol intake and the subsequent risk of stroke. What has been demonstrated is a J-shaped association between alcohol intake and stroke (Figure 7.1). Once again, moderate alcohol intake has protective effects, and is associated with a reduced risk of stroke compared with non-drinkers – and also compared with heavy drinkers. In contrast, high alcohol consumption (5 or more drinks daily) is associated with an increased risk of stroke.[155,156]

Does moderate alcohol intake increase your risk of cancer?

Alcohol is a carcinogen. A carcinogen is a chemical that causes cancer. It is well recognised that heavy alcohol consumption can increase the risk of all sorts of cancer – the most common being liver cancer and throat (laryngeal) cancer. What is less clear, but still crucially important, is whether moderate amounts of alcohol increase the risk of cancer. For most (but not all) cancers, there is no evidence that moderate alcohol has any effect on cancer risk. However, there is evidence that moderate alcohol increases the risk of cancer of the mouth, throat (oral and pharyngeal cancer), breast, liver and oesophagus.[157] Given the high rates of breast cancer in our population, this is certainly troubling. On the other hand, moderate alcohol appears to be protective with respect to the risk of certain other cancers – including kidney cancer and lymphoma.[158]

The Million Women Study[159] reported no increase in the risk of breast cancers in women having 3 or less drinks/week. But in women having 3–6 drinks per week, the rate of breast cancer increased slightly compared to non-drinkers, by about 8%. It is now well accepted that even small volumes of alcohol increase the risk of breast cancer in women. It also appears that there is a gradient of increasing risk with increasing alcohol intake.[160]

Alcohol and longevity

It's all well and good to say that a glass or 2 of wine a day will reduce my liver fat and my risk of heart attack and stroke, but how many more months or years of life do I get? The answer is impossible to know for any given individual, but statistically, moderate drinkers live on average, 2 years longer than non-drinkers. A number of studies have looked at this issue. Some report a survival advantage of more than 3 years, while others report as little as 6 months.[161,162] All the studies however, report that moderate drinkers live longer than non-drinkers.

One other very important piece of information gained from these reports relates to the quality of life of these extra years. The life-years gained by moderate drinkers are typically years of good health. I don't think any of us would care to spend an extra 2 years of life incapacitated, but if the extra years are spent in good health, then that is a significant gain.

It's also important to put the health benefits of moderate alcohol in context compared with other powerful public health messages such as exercise, stopping smoking and avoiding obesity. Of these issues, the one that exerts the greatest effect in terms of life-years gained is to avoid or stop smoking. Non-smokers live on average about 6 years longer than smokers. Regular exercise offers a survival benefit of about 3 years, while avoiding obesity adds an extra 12 months.[161]

When considered like this, some data suggests that moderate alcohol intake is perhaps two- or three-fold more powerful as a lifestyle choice to increase longevity than avoiding obesity. The lifestyle measures discussed here are generally additive in their effect on longevity. For example, a non-smoking, regular exerciser who drinks moderately and isn't obese lives between 8 and 15 years longer on average than their counterpart who smokes, doesn't exercise, doesn't drink and is obese.[161]

Live longer

Don't smoke – add an extra 6 years

Exercise – add an extra 3 years

Drink moderately – add an extra 1–3 years

Avoid obesity – add an extra year

Alcohol and all those calories

Alcohol is extremely calorie-dense. There are more calories in a gram of alcohol than there is in either a gram of protein or a gram of sugar. You would expect therefore that alcohol would cause weight gain. Perhaps surprisingly, no such evidence exists. We have previously discussed that weight gain is not necessarily related to calories; it depends on the hormonal response your body has to the food – primarily, the insulin response. A large insulin response to food typically results in weight gain, a small insulin response doesn't. Alcohol is an insulin-sensitiser, it makes your body more sensitive to insulin and lowers overall insulin levels.

Now how do you prove alcohol doesn't cause significant weight gain? The ideal design of a study to explore this would be to give one group of people a glass of wine with dinner and another group a glass of mineral water and see what happened to the weight of the 2 groups over a couple of years. Well, that trial has already been performed. Eighty people (all non-drinkers at the start of the study) were split into 3 groups. One group was assigned a glass of mineral water (no calories) with dinner, the next group, a glass of red wine (about 120 calories) and the final group, a glass of white wine (about 120 calories). The subjects were followed for the next 2 years. The individuals randomised to wine consumed an extra 12,480 calories compared with the water drinkers. At the end of the 2-year study, the red wine drinkers had gained less weight than the water drinkers.[163] Whether this phenomenon is true for beer and spirits is unclear at this stage.[164]

Evidence of the highest order

The gold-standard of trial design in medical research relies on data linking cause and effect – the randomised controlled trial. This involves taking 2 groups of people with similar characteristics and assigning one group to one therapy (or drug) and the other group another. At the conclusion of the study period, the effect of the intervention is measured. This may be an effect on liver function, blood pressure or survival, depending on what the trial is designed to explore.

The next 2 studies I discuss adhere to this trial design. These large randomised controlled trials have explored the potential beneficial metabolic effects of moderate alcohol intake in people with diabetes and its potential effect on their cholesterol and blood sugar.

In the first study, 224 non-drinking diabetics were assigned to either mineral water (the control group), 150 ml of white wine or 150 ml of red wine with dinner. The participants had their cholesterol, blood pressure and weight measured at the start of the study and regularly checked during the 2 years of the project. At the conclusion of the study the results showed a significant reduction in total cholesterol and an increase in good cholesterol in the red wine drinkers, compared to the other 2 groups.[163] The second study had a similar design and looked at the effect of moderate alcohol on blood pressure but found no real effect.[165]

So far, these are the largest randomised controlled trials examining the potential health benefits associated with moderate alcohol intake. Unfortunately, liver markers weren't examined in either of these trials.

Which type of alcoholic drink has the greatest health benefits?

We don't know everything, but from the existing data, all types of alcoholic drinks are associated with potentially positive health benefits, with the proviso that they are consumed in moderation. When all alcoholic drinks are compared however, red wine appears to be associated with slightly greater health benefits. The superiority of red wine may be due to resveratrol, which is found in high concentrations in red wine. As we discussed earlier, resveratrol is associated with multiple physiological benefits; it is an anti-inflammatory, anti-thrombotic and antioxidant.[166] It inhibits damage to blood vessel walls and reduces the risk of heart disease and/or stroke. Resveratrol also reduces the oxidation of fat that causes it to deposit itself on blood vessel walls, and reduces blood clot formation on top of these fat deposits (the process that initiates a heart attack).[163,165,167]

The liver is surprisingly resilient to regular alcohol intake. Even with heavy drinking, it takes in the order of 10 years or more before someone develops cirrhosis. Cirrhosis of the liver is not just dependent on the amount of alcohol you drink. Many heavy drinkers never develop cirrhosis (just like not all smokers develop lung disease); it is likely therefore that there are individual genetic factors that place some people at greater risk than others.

Alcohol-free days – do they help?

Does the liver need some non-drinking days to give it time to recover? Many people believe it does. The phenomenon of alcohol-free days has become so much part of our culture that it's got its own acronym, AFD. Even Feb Fast, or Dry July, when people stop drinking for the duration of February/July has been embraced by some as a health panacea. But does it do you any good? Does our liver need time off from alcohol? If our gut bacteria are producing alcohol 24/7, does it make any sense to stop drinking a couple of days per week?

To answer this question, we need data. We have data that compares the risk of premature death – from all causes – in non-drinkers, moderate drinkers and heavy drinkers. That data reveals that moderate drinkers have lower all-cause mortality than non-drinkers. Interestingly, when the moderate drinkers are divided into groups depending on how many days per week they drink, the greatest reduction in the risk of dying occurs in moderate drinkers who drank between 3 and 6 days per week. In essence, being a moderate drinker who has between 1 and 4 AFDs a week, gives you a further 5–10% reduction in the risk of premature death compared to moderate drinkers who drink every day.[168]

Other studies have reported similar findings; those with the greatest reduction in the risk of dying are moderate drinkers who have some alcohol-free days every week. Why we seem to benefit from AFDs is unclear, but there's a proven scientific benefit. As Mark Twain once quipped, 'Everything in moderation', including moderation.

The occasional binge

You may think that if you don't drink during the week you can save up and have your week's quota all together on a Friday or Saturday night. Don't be tempted. Binge drinking, or drinking alcohol with the specific intention of getting drunk, typically leads to alcohol-induced harm. Having more than 4 standard drinks at one sitting for women, or 5 for men, has negative social consequences such as increased risk of trauma, traffic accidents and violence. And for your liver, repeated episodes of binge drinking are detrimental and associated with a marked increase in the risk of developing cirrhosis. Binging also appears to have specific detrimental effects on heart health and is associated with an increased risk of death from heart disease.[169]

The hangover

'The delayed after-effects of drinking too much alcohol over a short period of time, characterised by headache and sometimes nausea and dizziness.' I've been there, and I guess you have too. Not the best feeling, is it? Modern science can explain the existence of dark matter, fly a space probe past Pluto and cure some cancers, but we still don't really know exactly what causes a hangover. Some scientists suggest a hangover is a manifestation of alcohol withdrawal – hence the premise of 'hair of the dog', with the implication being that the best treatment is to have another alcoholic drink. There is scientific evidence supporting this for some hangover symptoms but it doesn't tell the whole story.[170] A second hypothesis is that a hangover is caused by the accumulation of a toxic metabolite that forms after alcohol is broken down – acetaldehyde. Although high concentrations of this chemical can induce some symptoms of a hangover (sweating, flushing, nausea and vomiting), most of the acetaldehyde has been eliminated from the body by the time the hangover occurs.

A third hypothesis is that a hangover, at least in part, is caused by low blood sugar levels, resulting in nausea, tiredness, irritability and headaches. In a European study on blood sugar levels and alcohol, Dr Vartia[171] explored this hypothesis on 53 'volunteers' who had been apprehended for drunkenness. He tested their blood sugar on the night of their arrest, and again the following morning when they had sobered up. He also tested a control group who hadn't been drinking.

When they were drunk, the participants' blood sugar was elevated, but the following day when they were hung-over, the readings were significantly lower compared to those in the control group who hadn't been drinking. Vartia also found, the worse the hangover, the lower the blood sugar level. Interestingly, a Chinese medicine called KSS formula – containing plant compounds and brown sugar – has been shown in clinical studies to significantly reduce hangover severity. Perhaps the brown sugar resolves the low blood sugar aspect of the hangover.[172] This theory also fits nicely with your craving for a burger and coke the next morning.

One final hypothesis implicates the toxic effects of some chemicals in alcoholic drinks. The term *congeners* refers to minor chemical constituents in alcoholic drinks, which contribute to the drink's physiological effects. Congeners may include amines, amides, acetones, polyphenols, methanol and histamine. Some scientists blame the level of congeners in different drinks as the culprit contributing to a hangover. That might explain why some alcoholic drinks such as red wine, whisky and cognac (which are typically high in congeners) are more likely to produce a hangover than low congener drinks such as vodka and gin.[173]

It is likely that hangovers result from a combination of these factors rather than a single cause. As Joris Verster explained in a 2010 review of the treatment and prevention of the hangover: '(1) no effective hangover cures exist, (2) the scientific community lacks interest in examining hangover cures, and (3) the single effective way to prevent alcohol hangover is to moderate alcohol consumption'.[174]

A hangover after drinking means you are drinking too much. Some people experience hangover symptoms after as little as 2–3 drinks. Although this fits within the range we have discussed as moderate drinking, if you develop any hangover symptoms after drinking alcohol it is fair to suggest that this is your body saying, 'cut back'.

Alcohol and polyuria

Does alcohol make you urinate more? Conventional wisdom suggests it does. As we know however, conventional wisdom isn't always correct. So, what does science say about this? Maurice B Strauss and colleagues from the Cushing Veterans Hospital in Framingham, Massachusetts looked into this in 1950. Here, Strauss beautifully describes his experiment:

> 'The subjects, healthy adults, unaccustomed to the intemperate use of strong drink, were volunteers. They ate their breakfast ... and ... urine was passed as desired until 10.15 ... At 12.15 pm the bladder was again emptied ... and within a period of 4 to 6 minutes, 147 ml of 86 proof Bourbon whiskeys was ingested'.

Strauss gave 3 subjects 147 ml of whisky (50 g of alcohol) and another 3 subjects 147 ml of water and then measured the urine output of the 2 groups. No prize for guessing what happened. Alcohol made them urinate more. This excessive loss of water in urine contributes to the dehydration experienced during a hangover. However, the amount of excess water lost is perhaps surprising. Participants in the experiment lost about 600 ml of extra urine compared to those who drank water. This is about 120 ml of water lost for every 10 g of alcohol. Remembering that 10 g of alcohol is a standard drink, this means that for every standard drink, your body needs 120 ml of extra water, above and beyond your normal intake.

Drinking alcohol with meals is your best bet

Drinking with meals offers particular health advantages.[175,176] Indeed, some argue that drinking at other times means we forgo the potential health benefits typically assigned to moderate drinking.[177] Exactly how or why drinking with meals is good for you is hard to define; perhaps food slows the absorption of alcohol, which mimics the trickle of alcohol from our microbiome; or the antioxidative properties in wine may minimise damage to sensitive blood vessels from fats and other potentially hazardous compounds in meals.[177] Regardless of why, this seems advice worth taking.

Alcohol and adolescents

Children and adolescents are not just small adults – they are different. And all the studies done on the health benefits of alcohol have been done on adults, and therefore only apply to adults. There is now a vast amount of data suggesting alcohol use by children and young adults may adversely affect the developing brain and is a risk factor for alcohol problems later in life. As a result, there is no safe level for drinking in children and adolescents, and society and families should attempt to delay the initiation into drinking culture for as long as possible.

How big is a glass?

It has been well recognised for many years that serving size, including larger tableware increases consumption of food and non-alcoholic drinks, but up until recently, there has been no data describing whether this effect exists when it comes to alcohol drinking behaviour.

List of annual alcohol consumption per capita (litres of pure alcohol drunk)[178]

1	Belarus	17.5
2	Russia	15.1
3	Portugal	12.9
4	Poland	12.5
5	Finland	12.3
6	Australia	12.2
7	United Kingdom	11.6
8	Greece	10.3
9	United States	9.2
10	India	4.3

Over a 16-week period in 2015, the publican at The Pint Shop in Cambridge, England altered the size of glasses of wine he served in every fortnight to examine whether this affected wine sales.[179] He started with a standard wine glass (300 ml) then changed to a larger glass (370 ml), and then a smaller one (250 ml). The amount of wine poured into the glass remained the same (regardless of the glass size), but what changed was the perception of drinkers as to how much they were getting. The change in glass size made the volume of wine appear smaller (when the glass was larger) or larger with a smaller glass. Bigger glasses encouraged people to drink more because they felt there was a smaller volume of wine in the glass, leading them to drink faster and order more.

My recommendations . . .

The scientific evidence surrounding moderate alcohol intake and health is not totally resolved. I, personally, am a believer that moderate alcohol offers net benefits to a person's health but there are many others in the scientific community who interpret the data differently. This scientific contention primarily surrounds the interpretation of results from case control studies. These are studies that interview people about their alcohol intake and then examine potential associations with health outcomes. These studies clearly show that drinking heavily is associated with a wide variety of adverse outcomes. They also show that the more you drink the more likely these health consequences. The debate regarding moderate alcohol and health relates to the definitions of non-drinkers. We know that moderate drinkers have better liver function and better general health than non-drinkers. However, not all non-drinkers are the same. For example, people who have poor health may become non-drinkers for health reasons and that may explain some of the reason why moderate drinkers are, on average, healthier than non-drinkers. To overcome this potential confounder other studies have divided non-drinkers into lifetime non-drinkers and recent non-drinkers.

Studies with this design may utilise data from lifetime abstainers, which form the ideal control group. Most, but not all, studies that employ this design conclude that moderate alcohol offers net health benefits compared to lifetime abstaining.[180]

There's a term in astronomy known as 'the Goldilocks zone'. The Goldilocks zone is the region around a star where planets are at just the right temperature to have liquid water. Not so hot that all the water is burnt off, and not so cold that the water is frozen, but just right. It's the Goldilocks zone that you need to find for yourself when it comes to your alcohol consumption. A glass of wine at Christmas probably isn't enough to reap the metabolic benefits that moderate alcohol intake has been associated with. In contrast, more than 2 (for women) or 3 (for men) standard drinks a day, intermittent binging or experiencing hangovers means you drink too much. If, however, you have a glass of wine with your evening meal 3, 4 or even 5 nights a week, you are definitely in the Goldilocks zone.

Chapter 8

Liver tonics

The use of complementary and alternative medicine is absolutely booming. According to some reports, more than 60% of Australians say they have used complementary and alternative medicine (CAM) in the last year.[181] Estimates of spending on these therapies is in the order of $4 billion annually.[182] Some social researchers think this isn't a new thing, but that mainstream acceptance of alternative therapies now means it is okay to admit it.

One of the reasons people go looking for their own health answers beyond their GP's clinic is that Western medicine has real deficits when it comes to many concerns such as stress, pain and other symptoms that don't point to an easy diagnosis. People are also looking to play a more active role in their own health and longevity. This interest is spurred by the proliferation of books and articles promoting certain approaches involving specific foods and supplements as both life changing, and life-saving. The problem though, is while many natural remedies offer proven benefits, some are ineffective, and others are potentially dangerous. With vast profits up for grabs, people trying to help themselves can be vulnerable to falsehoods, shoddy quality control or well-meaning types who don't understand that even 'good' remedies won't work for everyone or are dangerous when taken with certain other supplements or medications.

Liver health is no exception. There are now innumerable products available that claim to augment liver health, detoxify the liver or treat liver-specific ailments. Let's take a look at what the science says.

Milk thistle

Milk thistle has been used as a herbal therapy for liver ailments for thousands of years. It goes by many names, including blessed thistle, Mark thistle, Marian thistle, Saint Mary's thistle, Mediterranean milk thistle, variegated thistle and Scotch thistle. It's an annual or biennial plant, growing up to 1.5 m tall and native to Southern Europe and Asia. The milk thistle extract used in herbal therapy is made from the seeds of the plant, which contain the compound silymarin.

Historically, milk thistle has been pitched as a therapy for all sorts of ailments, including warding off snakebite, irregular menstruation, to promote the flow of urine, clean the blood or improve the flow of bile. Over more recent times, milk thistle has become the most commonly prescribed herbal therapy for people suffering from any sort of liver complaint. Milk thistle has several metabolic effects on the liver. It acts as an antioxidant, reduces inflammation and affects several of the liver's metabolic pathways. It is generally thought to be a safe herbal therapy and negative side effects are uncommon, though they may include mild gastro-intestinal complaints such as bloating, diarrhoea and nausea.

But what about the science? There are hundreds of publications exploring milk thistle's potential role in promoting liver health. These studies generally involve small numbers of participants, and owing to the small numbers, it is hard to draw definitive conclusions. To help resolve this issue of small sample size, scientists analyse the pooled results of multiple studies on a given topic. The most prestigious and highly regarded of these reviews are those performed by Cochrane, a British charity formed to analyse medical research findings so as to facilitate evidence-based decision-making by health professionals. Publications from the Cochrane organisation are weighty and highly regarded. In fact, its publications specialise in reviews where data from a large number of trails is pooled to look for reliable outcomes. So, we're in luck that Cochrane has published a review specifically exploring the potential effect of milk thistle on liver health.

The Cochrane review explored the data relating to the use of milk thistle to treat liver disease from alcohol excess, hepatic B or hepatitis C. The review concluded that milk thistle had no effect on reducing the death rate from liver disease in these patient groups.[183] The review noted that milk thistle had a minor effect on improving some liver function tests. Overall, the Cochrane review was disappointing with respect to any potential positive health effect of the herb in these conditions.

Another review published in 2014 nicely summarised the studies exploring the use of milk thistle in people with fatty liver disease.[184] The herb appears to be associated with positive metabolic effect when used for fatty liver disease, including improvements in liver function tests and liver fat, and also improved insulin sensitivity. Reviewed data from nearly 600 people with fatty liver disease enrolled in eight separate trials concluded that the herb was associated with positive and significant[185] improvements in liver function tests.[184]

In my opinion, the data relating to milk thistle is strong enough that it can be considered of benefit when it comes to liver health. It's also important to note that there was no suggestion in any of the studies that milk thistle resulted in any harm to people.

The death cap mushroom and milk thistle

The death cap mushroom (amanita phalloides) grows around the base of oak trees, and contains a toxin that damages liver cells.

It is extremely poisonous, with as little as half a mushroom being enough to kill an adult. Typically, a couple of days after consuming the death cap, symptoms of liver failure (jaundice, confusion) develop rapidly and people can die within hours or days.

Milk thistle extract in treating wild mushroom poisoning

A 71-year-old man saw his doctor after he developed nausea, vomiting and severe diarrhoea. Initial blood tests revealed evidence of severe liver injury. The visit to the doctor was 2 days after a meal of wild mushrooms while camping in Iowa.

The patient was transferred to a large city hospital where his condition deteriorated, and he became confused (a manifestation of life-threatening liver failure). The patient was then given an infusion of milk thistle extract. Over the next few days the patient's liver injury improved and the man was discharged from hospital,[186] going on to make a full recovery.

While this is not scientific proof of the liver benefits of milk thistle, there is increasing evidence that milk thistle may minimise liver injury in death cap mushroom poisoning. Indeed, it has now become part of the standard care at many medical centres in Australia and Europe.[187]

Curcumin (turmeric)

Curcumin is one of the components of turmeric, which has been used in traditional Chinese medicine to treat a variety of ailments from acne and arthritis to cancer for thousands of years. More recently, it has become widely available in Western countries as a supplement and a tea. It has been touted as being anti-inflammatory and antioxidative, and has featured in small medical trials for a variety of conditions.

So far we don't have a great deal of scientific data on its use in humans, although the data we do have suggests curcumin may well be a promising agent for people with fatty liver disease. Curcumin has primarily been studied for diabetes treatment, and as we know from earlier chapters, diabetes and liver health are often interrelated because of the shared mechanism of insulin resistance. In these studies, curcumin appears to reduce appetite, reduce total body fat and visceral fat (the bad fat).[188] Thus, if these early studies can be repeated and performed in people with fatty liver disease, it may well become an important agent.

Unfortunately, the current data is insufficient to advocate its use. There have been no good-quality studies that explore its role in liver health generally or any potential role in treating liver disease.[189] What you can do though, is add turmeric to your cooking occasionally, or even order a turmeric latte now and then.

Dandelion leaf extract (taraxacum)

Dandelion leaf extract is a common compound in many 'liver tonics' sold in health food shops. There is some science suggesting beneficial effects of this compound on the livers of rodents, but not in humans. If you are a mouse with liver disease it may be something you should nibble on. For us humans however, there is no evidence of any benefit as yet.

What is interesting about dandelion leaf, is that it was often included as a part of the traditional Mediterranean diet, which included foraged wild greens such as dandelion leaf and arugula. These bitter leaves may just add an extra something to your next salad.

Barberry (berberis vulgaris)

Despite claims by some supplement companies that this compound has been traditionally used in Western medicine for liver support, there is very little published human data to support its role in liver health. Although one small study suggested barberry may improve liver function test results in fatty liver disease,[190] currently there is not enough data in Western medicine literature to suggest it is of benefit.

Artichoke leaf extract (cynara)

Once again, although this compound is touted as a liver protective agent within the alternative medicine world, there is little scientific data to support the claim. In fact, one study of its use in patients with hepatitis C showed it was no better than a placebo.[191]

Schisandra

Schisandra is a red berry native to China and Russia, used to promote liver health in traditional medicine. Maybe it does some good – but that's the best we can say right now. There is only a small amount of human data suggesting it may help improve liver tests in some people.[192]

Vitamin A

Carotenoids are the chemical precursor to vitamin A and are present in many red and orange vegetables, most famously, of course, the carrot. It has been demonstrated that the more carotenoids you have in your diet, the healthier your liver is. But while it may seem a reasonable conclusion that vitamin A supplementation will offer liver health benefits, let's look at the evidence. The recommended intake of vitamin A for adults is in the order of 700-900 ug per day. Many vitamin preparations however, contain well above the recommended daily intake. Taking one or 2 vitamin A capsules a day is not uncommon, but this may provide individuals with more than 10 times the recommended daily allowance.[193] It's too much.

The dangers of high dose vitamin A supplements

In 2007, a 59-year-old man sought medical attention with symptoms of liver failure.[194] He consulted his local doctor after gradually developing a swollen abdomen over the preceding 6 months. On examination, the doctor discovered the patient's abdomen was swollen with fluid as a consequence of liver failure. X-rays demonstrated the patient had cirrhosis. His liver blood tests were significantly abnormal.

The patient described taking over-the-counter vitamin supplements for the last 2 years containing a daily intake of 13,000 ug of vitamin A – fifteen times the recommended level. Extensive investigations were undertaken to identify any other causes of the patient's liver failure and none were identified. He was advised to stop taking the vitamin supplements immediately. Over the next 2 years the patient's condition gradually improved.

This is not a one-off case! There are numerous reports of vitamin A overdoses, many with exposure to doses much lower than the patient just discussed.[195] One of the most notorious stories associated with vitamin A poisoning had nothing to do with modern supplements and involved a torturous and deadly trek in Antarctica.

Sir Douglas Mawson arrived in Commonwealth Bay Antarctica in January 1912 with the aim of exploring and mapping the continent. Several teams on sleds pulled by huskies went off in different directions. Mawson travelled with Xavier Mertz and Belgrave Ninnis.

After many weeks of exploration, the party was nearly 500 km from base camp when Ninnis fell through a crevasse, taking the 6 best dogs with him, as well as the team's tent and most of their rations. Ninnis died, and following a brief service, Mawson and Mertz turned immediately for base camp. With little food, the pair were forced to use several of their remaining dogs as sustenance for themselves and the other dogs. Over the 13 days following the accident, 6 dogs were killed and eaten – including their livers, which of course are extremely high in vitamin A. 'It was a happy relief when the liver appeared, even if little else could be said in its favour, it was easily chewed and demolished' (Mawson's diary). Two days later, the weather turned and the explorers decided to rest. Soon after Mertz developed severe dysentery and became depressed.

At the same time, both Mertz and Mawson suffered classic symptoms of vitamin A toxicity. Both men experienced peeling skin and hair loss. The skin on Mawson's ears came off in casts. Both lost all the skin from their genitals and legs. Mertz died soon after, while Mawson slowly made it back to base camp, arriving about 4 weeks later weighing just 51 kg, compared to his normal 95 kg. His story of survival is one of the greatest in the era of Antarctic exploration. Although there is some debate[196] many attribute the death of Mertz to vitamin A poisoning from eating the liver of the sled dogs.[197]

Vitamin A cannot be advocated as a liver protective agent or as a therapeutic agent in people with liver disease. Vitamin A supplements, especially in high doses, may cause liver disease or worsen pre-existing liver problems and should be avoided![198]

Vitamin C

Which species cannot synthesise their own vitamin C? The answer? Bats, guinea pigs, capybaras (otherwise known as the world's largest rodents), and us. So, we humans are one of the few species that need vitamin C in our diet to prevent disease.

Vitamin C supports the immune system, and supplements are often used to treat and ward off colds. It is also essential for several chemical reactions, including the synthesis of collagen. Collagen is one of the principal building blocks for all our structural tissues. It exists, at a microscopic level, as bands of fibrous tissue that make up our bones, tendons, ligaments and skin. Inadequate levels of vitamin C result in scurvy. The symptoms of scurvy are primarily related to an inability to make enough collagen – including spongy bleeding gums, fragile spotty skin and eventually, open wounds, loss of teeth and death.

Apart from vitamin C's impact on collagen synthesis and the immune system, it is also an antioxidant and reduces inflammation in tissues. For this latter reason, its role in liver disease has been explored due to its potential to reduce inflammation and scarring.

Vitamin C supplements are not recommended for anyone with liver disease, unless the patient has a dietary deficiency.[199] The information available suggests vitamin C doesn't offer any benefits for liver disease, or people wanting to augment liver health. There is even some suggestion that vitamin C supplements are associated with an increased risk of liver cancer.[200] One enormous Chinese study collected data on diet and supplements in more than 132,000 individuals and examined their subsequent risk of developing liver cancer. In this study, the authors revealed a higher risk of cancer in those taking vitamin C supplements, but not in those whose vitamin C came from dietary sources.

Vitamin D

If we're getting all semantic, then vitamin D isn't even a vitamin, it's a hormone. The term vitamin refers to an essential chemical that is ingested from food. As we all know, vitamin D is synthesised in our skin from exposure to sunlight, specifically UVB radiation. In humans, almost all of our vitamin D is synthesised with only small amounts contributed by our diet. Dietary sources of vitamin D include oily fish (salmon, tuna, mackerel and sardines), mushrooms and alfalfa.

The primary role of vitamin D in humans is to aid the absorption of calcium and other minerals from the small intestine. This means, long-term vitamin D deficiency can result in inadequate calcium absorption, leading to reduced bone strength, and in the worst cases, rickets in children and osteomalacia in adults. Vitamin D is also increasingly recognised for the important role it plays in our immune system, and deficiency during childhood is believed to be a significant factor in the subsequent development of multiple sclerosis (MS) and numerous other diseases.

The relationship between sunshine exposure, vitamin D and liver disease is not yet crystal clear, but it appears that a lack of sunshine and/or a lack of vitamin D is detrimental to the liver. It has now been clearly demonstrated that the lower your vitamin D levels, the more likely you are to have fatty liver disease and the more likely your fatty liver disease is to be severe.[201] With our modern lifestyle, a lot of time is spent indoors. This phenomenon explains why vitamin D deficiency is becoming increasingly common. In Australia, up to one third of adults are vitamin D deficient.[202] Vitamin D deficiency is more common in people at higher latitudes (further from the equator), older individuals, the overweight and in individuals with darker skin pigmentation.

There are a number of clinical studies investigating whether vitamin D supplements help fatty liver disease, but at present, none of these studies have been completed. Given how common vitamin D deficiency is, its role in bone disease and its potential role in a long list of other diseases it is reasonable to ask whether routine supplementation is safe. Vitamin D supplements reduce the risk of premature death in older individuals, by perhaps 10%.[203] In sensible doses (500–2000 IU daily), vitamin D supplementation appears extremely safe. In very high doses, supplementation potentially causes kidney damage and even kidney failure. For liver health, and your health in general, get sensible amounts of sun exposure and, if you can't, consider taking a vitamin D supplement. The amount of sun exposure that individuals require to maintain adequate vitamin D levels has created a confusing public health message because of the overlapping issue of sun exposure and skin cancer risk. In summer, 5–10 minutes of sun exposure on the face and arms each day is adequate for most people. In winter, it gets more problematic due to the angle of the sun at different latitudes. In tropical areas, even in winter, 5–10 minutes of sun daily remains adequate. In the middle latitudes (25–40 degrees) this increases to 15–30 minutes and in higher latitudes, more than 30 minutes of sun exposure a day is needed. Many people who live in the south of Australia won't be getting enough sun exposure in winter, so seasonal vitamin D augmentation remains a sensible option.

Foods high in vitamin D

- Liver
- Mushrooms
- Oily fish
- Dairy products (vitamin D is often added to milk)
- Soy milk (vitamin D is often added to soy milk)
- Caviar
- Eggs
- Fortified cereals

Vitamin E

Vitamin E refers to a group of eight similar fat-soluble compounds most often referred to as tocopherols. Vitamin E is primarily found in plant oils and acts as a natural antioxidant. In fatty liver disease patients, vitamin E has been shown to reduce inflammation, reduce liver fat, and also reduce liver damage seen on liver biopsy. The doses used in the studies on fatty liver disease were 800 IU daily.[204] As far as I'm aware, this is the only high-quality data in the published literature showing that any vitamin supplement is of clear benefit to people with liver disease. Following this data, vitamin E supplementation has become the mainstay of drug therapy for people with significant liver injury from fatty liver disease. But as with everything in life, the vitamin E supplement story is complicated.

As we have discussed in the chapters on alcohol, it's no use taking something that helps your liver if it causes serious consequences to you in other ways. This is my concern with vitamin E – it may help your liver, but do you harm elsewhere.

More than a decade ago, an enormous study was initiated in the United States to gauge whether the risk of prostate cancer could be reduced by long-term administration of either vitamin E or selenium supplements. More than 35,000 men were recruited for the study and were given a placebo, vitamin E or selenium; or both vitamin E and selenium.[205] It was found that the men given vitamin E supplements had a significantly increased rate of prostate cancer. For me, this means vitamin E can't be advocated as a routine treatment for fatty liver disease in men. The association between prostate cancer and vitamin E supplements remains important as a public health issue for men – especially as up to 50% of men over 60 are taking supplements containing vitamin E.[206] The dose of vitamin E used in the prostate cancer prevention trial was 400 IU daily, half the dose used in the fatty liver studies, but much higher than the recommended daily allowance of just 15 IU.[207]

The story surrounding vitamin E supplements gets even more concerning when we consider studies that suggest it increases all-cause mortality.[208] Peer reviewed published data suggests you are more likely to die prematurely if you take vitamin E supplements than if you don't!

Fish oil supplements

A diet high in fish is good for your health; the truth of this is now so well established that there is little debate surrounding it. A diet high in oily fish has been linked to reductions in heart disease, improved cognition, improvements in symptoms of rheumatoid arthritis and benefits for mental health too. A diet high in seafood also benefits liver health.[209]

The discussion, however, becomes less clear when we start to examine the science behind fish oil supplements for liver health and health in general. Fish oil is high in omega-3 fatty acids. Omega-3 fatty acids are essential polyunsaturated fatty acids that cannot be synthesised by the body. There are 2 main forms of omega-3 fatty acids, DHA and EPA. Several small studies suggest omega-3 fatty acids are beneficial for liver disease as their use has been shown to reduce liver fat and improve liver function, at least in some people with fatty liver disease.[210] The complexity in implementing this observation however is that the dose of fish oil needed to obtain the liver health benefits is very high. The dose used in one Japanese study was 2,700 mg of EPA, the active ingredient in fish oil.[211] Studies that have used smaller doses have generally been negative.[212] If you are going to take fish oil supplements to augment liver health, then check the dose on the bottle and make sure you take the dose associated with health benefits.

Probiotics

As we discussed in Chapter 3, probiotics are foods or supplements which contain live bacteria; whereas prebiotics are foods or food ingredients that promote the growth of beneficial bacteria in the gut – i.e. that feed the bacteria already in the gut. Synbiotics contain both probiotics and prebiotics.

Probiotics appear to be beneficial for liver health. A trial performed in 2014 in Iran involved 72 patients with fatty liver disease; half were asked to take 300 g of a probiotic yoghurt (containing lactobacillus and bifidobacterium), and the other half consumed 300 g of conventional yoghurt that contained no bacteria. At the end of the 8-week study period, subjects taking the probiotic yoghurt had improved liver blood tests, and lower cholesterol levels. No changes at all were observed in those eating the conventional yoghurt.[67] Other studies have replicated these findings with capsules containing different probiotic bacteria (lactobacillus and streptococcus).[213]

Another study explored the role of a commercially available probiotic preparation called VSL3; a mixture of 8 probiotic strains (streptococcus thermophilus, bifidobacteria [B. breve, B. infantis, B. longum], lactobacillus acidophilus, L. plantarum, L. paracasei, and L. delbrueckii subsp. bulgaricus). This Italian study, led by Dr Alisi, explored the role of VSL3 in children with fatty liver disease. Half the children were prescribed VSL3, and the other half a placebo. Dr Alisi demonstrated that at the end of a 4-month period, there was significant reduction in liver fat in the children taking the probiotic and also that their weight had also fallen. The weight loss suggests the probiotic has a systemic effect such that it changed the children's general metabolisms and not just their liver function.[214]

As suggested by Dr Alisi's trial, the beneficial effects of probiotics aren't just confined to the liver. Probiotics have now been shown to have a number of beneficial metabolic effects. They lower cholesterol, reduce body weight, reduce waist circumference, improve blood sugar control in diabetics and also lower markers of inflammation.[215] What we don't know, is whether the beneficial effects relate to one specific bacterial species or to a mix of different ones. We also don't know whether there is a specific dose associated with a maximum beneficial effect. What I can say is that the beneficial effects are observed with a wide variety of preparations that contain many different bacteria. It seems therefore that most commercial preparations make beneficial contributions.

At the checkout

If you are going to spend some of your hard-earned dollars on a commercial product to improve your liver health, then I suggest you buy something backed by science. For now, that's limited to fish oil (possibly, and only in high doses), probiotics and milk thistle (at a stretch). It is important to point out that just because a product is marketed as a natural or herbal product doesn't necessarily mean that it is gentle or benign. In some instances, herbal therapies can cause severe liver injury including life-threatening liver failure.[216,217]

Part 3

A better liver lifestyle

Chapter 9

Beyond the plate

Sitting down on the job and liver disease

One of the aims of this book is to dispel the myths regarding diet for liver health and good health in general. It is possible, after all, to eat an interesting diet, indulge in coffee, alcohol and chocolate, and despite that, have a healthy liver in a healthy body. But what about lying on the couch watching TV? There is no doubt that this is one of the joys of the modern world. What more could you wish for than relaxing on the couch, glass of red wine in one hand and a piece of chocolate in the other, watching TV and knowing you are looking after yourself?

Now I hope you are sitting down for this news. Hopefully this is the only downer you'll read in this book. The red wine and chocolate are fine. However, the sad reality is that lying on the couch watching TV is bad for you and your liver.[218] The more you watch, the more upset your liver is. It is unlikely that TV per se has any detrimental effect on the liver but there are well-documented associations between TV viewing and weight gain. Being overweight is strongly associated with excess visceral fat and the ensuing liver damage we've been talking about. Sorry to break the bad news to you, but sometimes a person needs to come out and tell it as it is. Humans have not evolved to be sitting or lying down for prolonged periods of time. This is a modern phenomenon and it's not good for us.

Prolonged sitting directly results in liver damage, and not just because of its potential association with reduced exercise. Our twenty-first century lifestyle sitting at a desk and tapping away on a computer, sitting in the car or on the train during our commute, followed by sitting on the couch to eat dinner and watch TV may be slowly killing us.

The evidence also directly links prolonged sitting with a variety of other life-threatening medical conditions including diabetes, cardiovascular disease, cancer and mental illness. Scientists from South Korea examined the impact of prolonged sitting on the risk of developing fatty liver disease, including whether prolonged sitting just resulted in reduced exercise and if the lack of exercise was the mechanism leading to liver damage. Referencing the health records of 140,000 Koreans who underwent health checks between 2011 and 2013,[219] the researchers found that prolonged sitting and reduced physical activity were both independently associated with developing fatty liver. The more time spent sitting, the more likely individuals were to develop liver disease. Another important and concerning finding of the Korean study was that sitting induced liver damage in people who were not overweight. Conventionally, fatty liver disease has been seen as a condition generally confined to people who are overweight or obese. What the Korean study identified, was that prolonged sitting itself leads to insulin resistance and all the associated adverse metabolic outcomes – even if you are lean.

Prolonged sitting induces liver damage. This effect can occur even if you exercise adequately and have a healthy body weight.

How moving helps your liver

Somehow it seems to be counter-intuitive to link exercise and liver health. I think we can all logically agree that exercise is of benefit to the health of our heart, lungs and muscles, but the liver? Yet it's real – exercise has dramatic effects on liver health. Although fatty liver disease is the most common liver disease, and indeed one of the most common medical conditions worldwide, it was only recognised as a distinct entity in 1980. Exercise, although it has become one of the mainstays of therapy for the condition, has only been recognised to have an effect on liver function as recently as 1990.[220]

In Chapter 3, I talked about the dial we all have that sets our metabolic profile. If this dial is turned too far to the right, we get elevated levels of insulin, develop liver fat and scarring, and are at risk of premature death from liver disease, heart disease and cancer. Exercise helps turn this metabolic dial in the healthy direction.

In people with liver fat, the standard advice from physicians is to exercise more and lose weight. We know that both of these measures improve liver health by reducing liver fat – but we also know that advising people to lose significant weight is almost futile. For many people reducing body weight by 5% or less is achievable, although it may be difficult. Losing more than this and keeping it off is extremely difficult. Generally, once you have gained weight, your body accepts this as the new normal and tries to maintain it. This is why most people who lose weight by dieting put it back on gradually in the following months or years.[221] The ineffectiveness of calorie restricted diets to control weight in the longer term is now so well recognised that medical negligence claims have been made against doctors for failure to refer obese patients for weight loss surgery or other specialist services.[222]

For a minute though, let's put aside the usual associations between exercise and weight loss. The fact is that even if you exercise without losing a single gram of body weight, there are significant health and well-being advantages to exercising. The scientific evidence shows exercise improves liver health in people with fatty liver even if they don't lose any weight because in and of itself, exercise reduces insulin levels and turns the metabolic dial back in the healthy direction.

Exercise – how much is enough?

It's surprising that science is only just now beginning to understand the effects of different forms of exercise on health. Public health recommendations typically advise the general population to undertake 30 minutes of moderate activity most days of the week. However, most of us fail to reach this target, with time cited as the biggest barrier.

However, recent data offers new hope to the time poor, suggesting we can achieve the physiological benefits exercise offers without the onerous time commitment. Dr Jamie Timmons led a research project in Edinburgh that involved 16 unfit young men.[223] He had them do 7 minutes of high intensity exercise per week, involving 4–6 repetitions of 30-second sprints on an exercise bicycle, repeated every second or third day. At the end of the 2 weeks of the study, participants showed marked reductions in insulin and glucose levels.

The details on how much exercise is necessary to reduce liver fat remains undefined. That some exercise is better than nothing is no doubt true. When explored scientifically, studies that have looked at whether high levels or low levels of exercise are necessary to achieve a reduction in liver fat have surprisingly found that the amount may not make much difference.[224] Similar results have also been demonstrated when exploring variations in intensity. High intensity and low intensity exercise appear to be equally beneficial for liver health.[224] Exercise and dietary modification are complementary interventions. Changing your diet to support your liver will dramatically aid health, as will increasing your exercise. The effect of changing diet in addition to increasing exercise is additive.

The benefits of diet and exercise are not mutually exclusive; they are complementary,[225] with the effect of diet and exercise together much greater than the effect of either alone.

The benefits from 'micro' exercising bring another long-held belief into focus. We have all been led to believe that when it comes to exercise, more is better. While that may be true to a point, for those of us who are mostly sedentary, the relationship between exercise and health is not linear. You can overdo exercise, even though the last 40 years has seen our culture embrace physical feats of endurance and the extreme athlete. Consider how the marathon has gone from an Olympic event to something regular people aspire to. Triathlons, which were once an exotic event undertaken in Hawaii, are now commonly held in many cities around the world and performed not just by mature adults but increasingly by children. This extreme commitment to pushing your physical boundaries suggests the psyche of our community has accepted that to achieve good health you must suffer. By implication, the more exercise we do, the better we are. How did we get to this?

When it's all too much

In 490 BC, Philippides was a messenger in the Greek army. Following a victory over the Persians on the battlefield, Philippides was dispatched from Marathon to Athens to announce the victory to the government. It is said he ran this distance without stopping. He burst into the Greek assembly announcing, 'We have won!' before falling to the floor and dying. The distance from the battlefield in Marathon to Athens was 25 miles and the legend of the run is the basis for the modern-day marathon. But Philippides died.

The scientific evidence we have is that very high-level physical activity may be just as bad for us as no activity at all. High-level exercise induces an extreme stress on the heart and is associated with disease in the heart arteries, structural damage to the heart and also increased incidence of sudden death.[226] So, while the average person will live longer if they exercise more, the argument and the evidence only holds so far. We now know that men and women performing high levels of regular exercise lose the protection from premature death that moderate exercise confers and are actually more likely to die than individuals performing low or moderate levels of exercise.[227]

Working out along a middle path

For many people exercise can appear to be another chore they just don't have the time or motivation to pursue. I can fully understand why people start running and then stop after 3 months, or join a gym and stop attending after 6 months – it is just too boring for many of us. Instead try to factor in enjoyment right from the start of a new regime. Why not go for a walk with a friend, play social tennis or join a basketball team? I run (jog, actually) with a friend and afterwards we sit down with a glass of wine and discuss the world's problems. It turns something that would otherwise be hard work into something to look forward to.

Evolution has designed us to take it easy

There is an obvious paradox when it comes to the health benefits of exercise. Decades of public health messages that have made it clear to us all that moderate levels of physical exercise are necessary to maintain our health. Despite this crystal-clear message, achieving this health-promoting level of exercise is beyond the majority of the population. Why is this? What could explain why most of us fail to act in our own self-interest when it comes to getting enough exercise? It's evolution. As the famous biologist Theodosius Dobzhansky quoted 50 years ago, 'Nothing in biology makes sense except in the light of evolution'.[228] As humans and all other living organisms evolved, rather than being designed, we need to consider evolutionary history to understand why we are the way we are.

Although humans have evolved as physically active athletes, we are just as adapted to being lazy and sedentary whenever possible. Evolution tells us to exercise only when absolutely necessary (to maintain adequate nutrition and ensure reproductive success) and also as play. There is no evolutionary reason to exercise when at least one of these 2 goals is not being met.

Getting into the rhythm of sleeping well

It has been recognised for many years that liver disease can cause sleep disturbance. Now there is also evidence that sleep disturbance may be a significant cause of liver disease, specifically contributing to fatty liver disease. This makes it more important than ever to take getting a good night's sleep seriously.

Melatonin, one of the primary hormones regulating our sleep/wake cycle, is released by the pineal gland, a very small protuberance on the base of the brain. This hormone makes you sleepy of an evening and signals your body that it's time for bed. Light, specifically blue light, inhibits the production of melatonin during the day and it is only when light levels begin to fall after sunset that melatonin production increases, leading to that sleepy feeling you get late of an evening. Unfortunately, lifestyle factors commonly disrupt this simple cycle. Once the sun sets, modern lighting such as overhead lights, TV and handheld screens all confuse our melatonin regulated sleep/wake cycle such that we can't get the full melatonin surge that nature designed. This leads to poor sleep initiation and poor sleep quality. It is the blue end of the light spectrum that most influences the pineal gland to inhibit melatonin release. However, many phones and laptops now have a mechanism to limit blue light at night, so the device causes less disruption to the sleep/wake cycle.

Sleep disturbance is very commonly seen in patients with cirrhosis. In people with this condition, the evening surge of melatonin may be disturbed causing the sleep/wake cycle to be delayed many hours. Patients may wander the house all night exhausted, but are unable to get off to sleep until the early hours of the morning.[229] They then sleep until well into the day. This dysfunctional sleep/wake cycle obviously impacts significantly on an individual's quality of life.

The circadian rhythm that regulates the sleep/wake cycle, making you feel mentally bright during the day and sleepy of an evening, also regulates chemical reactions in your liver. During daylight hours when we eat, our liver nutrient metabolism and detoxification pathways are ramped up. These systems then reduce their efficiency during the evening and night – which is when we have evolved to be fasting. With sleep disturbance there is dysregulation of liver enzyme activity and feeding/fasting cycle, contributing to elevated insulin secretion and fatty liver injury.[230]

Ignoring or disrupting the circadian rhythm interferes with liver function, because fasting overnight is important for the liver enzymes to do their thing. Eating late increases insulin secretion and fatty liver injury.

What else could be blocking your sleep?

In Western society the most common disorder affecting sleep is obstructive sleep apnoea. Obstructive sleep apnoea affects approximately 25–35% of obese individuals. It is most often characterised by loud frequent snoring and excessive daytime tiredness. In individuals with obstructive sleep apnoea, there are multiple repeated periods during sleep where breathing ceases for many seconds to minutes. During these periods the throat collapses blocking the flow of air and patients repeatedly wake to open the throat and allow airflow to resume.

It may come as no surprise at all that obese individuals with obstructive sleep apnoea may also have fatty liver disease, but the scientific evidence says that the 2 conditions are related not just by the shared risk factor of obesity. Obstructive sleep apnoea, by itself, contributes to insulin resistance. There is also evidence that treatment of obstructive sleep apnoea improves liver function, suggesting obstructive sleep apnoea and fatty liver are cause and effect, not just association. In one study of 40 obese men with obstructive sleep apnoea, treatment (with a nasal mask worn overnight), resulted in a marked reduction in ALT levels, and this was maintained in the long term.[231] The hypothesis on how obstructive sleep apnoea results in liver injury is that the low levels of oxygen in the blood overnight in these patients results in liver damage and fat accumulation.

Even more interestingly, poor sleep by itself may lead to fatty liver disease, even in people without obesity or obstructive sleep apnoea. One Korean study assessed sleep duration and quality in 69,000 middle aged workers and their spouses and explored the relationship with liver disease. In both sexes, poor quality sleep was associated with the presence of fatty liver even when the data was adjusted for the traditional fatty liver risk factors of obesity and diabetes. Sleep duration less than 5 hours was a risk factor for developing fatty liver disease.[232] Several other studies have now reported similar findings.[233]

It appears that inadequate sleep induces the accumulation of pathogenic liver fat via a number of mechanisms. Sleep deprivation elevates levels of chemicals in the blood that go on to cause liver injury; these are called pro-inflammatory cytokines.[234] Sleep deprivation also stimulates the hormones that control appetite and reduces the hormones controlling satiety.[235] Thus, poor sleep can fuel weight gain. One especially interesting hypothesis linking poor sleep and fatty liver involves the adrenal glands and secretion of the stress hormone cortisol.

If you are chronically tired, it changes your hormone levels, making you feel hungrier and less satisfied.

Can stress contribute to liver disease?

Hopefully I have convinced you by now that a broad, tasty diet, coffee, exercise and sleep can also facilitate liver health. But your stress levels also matter. A 2016 study from China explored this specific issue. Dr Chen Li and colleagues interviewed more than 2,000 police officers, to understand the relationship between work-related stress and fatty liver disease.[236] Overall, one third of the officers had fatty liver. Moderate or high levels of occupational stress and also high levels of personal strain were associated with the development of fatty liver. This relationship persisted even after adjusting for age, body weight and levels of exercise; all the traditional factors that may contribute to fatty liver disease. Obviously, association does not prove causation, but prospective controlled trials are difficult to design and administer in the area of work-related stress.

One very important piece of the puzzle that ties together stress and liver disease is outlined in a paper published in 2015 in the prestigious medical journal *Gastroenterology*.[237] This project was led by Tom Russ from the Division of Psychiatry, University of Edinburgh. The paper was a meta-analysis; it pooled the data from a number of smaller publications that had explored the area of liver-related mortality and psychological distress. Psychological distress was measured using a questionnaire that explored symptoms of anxiety, depression, social dysfunction and loss of confidence. Overall, the researchers analysed data from 166,600 individuals. Their analysis revealed that individuals with the highest levels of psychological distress were 3.5 times more likely to die from liver disease than those with low levels of distress. It is possible that those with the most distress also drank excess alcohol and were overweight. Tom Russ and team then adjusted the data for these confounders and still found that death from liver disease was much more common in people with greater levels of stress. There was also a strong association between the levels of stress and liver-related mortality, a finding that helps support the premise that stress and liver disease are related by cause and effect not just by chance.

Chronic sleep deprivation and long-term psychological stress both cause similar pathological changes to human physiology. Levels of inflammatory chemicals in the blood are elevated, appetite-stimulating hormones are induced and the adrenal glands of the body are stimulated in a flight or fight response to release the stress hormone cortisol.

Cortisol

The adrenal glands are small fat-containing organs that sit on top of the kidneys. Their main role is to secrete steroid hormones that are involved in a variety of bodily functions. Of the most importance to us is cortisol. Cortisol is one of the primary hormones involved in the flight or fight response. It prepares the body for life-threating events.

Cortisol facilitates the release of glucose into the blood to provide fuel for muscles. From an evolutionary viewpoint, this allows us to run away from predators. This short-term surge in cortisol is an appropriate and life-saving physiological response.

The problems begin when the cortisol fails to drop off again after an initial surge. In our complicated modern lives, we are exposed to non-stop stimuli that lead to regular and more prolonged cortisol secretion. Driving to work in traffic, running late for meetings, financial stress, health concerns for our children, workplace dissatisfaction and sleep deprivation all stimulate the flight and fight response – in an ongoing fashion. The result is that cortisol levels, instead of surging just occasionally, are chronically elevated. This long-term elevation in cortisol levels contributes to fat deposition, insulin resistance and fatty liver disease.

One 2015 study involving 17 healthy men and women with sleep deprivation resulted in significant elevation in cortisol levels the following day. The sleep deprivation also increased stress ratings in the subjects.[238] Similar findings have also been reported, with workplace stress elevating cortisol levels in teachers and other professionals.[239,240] Elevated levels of cortisol have also been clearly associated with the development and progression of fatty liver disease.[241] Given these clear associations between modern lifestyle, cortisol elevations and fatty liver, stress-reducing lifestyle interventions seem appropriate for us all. Exercise, social engagement, laughter, mindfulness and meditation are all associated with reduction in cortisol levels.

Part 4

Go forth and flourish

Chapter 10

Liver better life

Liver health is central to your well-being. Liver dysfunction is the canary in the coalmine signalling that your lifestyle choices may be the harbinger of both your liver's downfall and an elevated risk of death from cardiac disease, diabetes and a wide range of cancers.

I'm fine, you may think. But if you are over 40, and even slightly overweight, you're at significant risk, and as we've discussed, there's that phenomenon of being thin on the outside and fat on the inside. You might not be able to see it, but the visceral fat you are carrying around your organs is conspiring to kill you.

My aim in writing this book has been to present evidence-based information to empower people to take control of their liver health and live well. One of the remarkable attractions of the *liver better* lifestyle is that living well and enjoying pleasurable foods is good for you.

But making the best choices for your liver and overall health also comes with an understanding that our bodies, motivations and hormones evolved in an environment in which scarcity was the norm. For most Westerners, we need to find ways to 'sit comfortably' with being hungry sometimes – to understand that we don't need to react to every prompt to reach for a snack, and to choose foods that are unprocessed rather than the highly sweetened modern options that send us into a craving spiral.

Find ways to 'sit comfortably' with being hungry sometimes – we don't need to react to every prompt to reach for a snack.

The 1970s saw the first data linking lifestyle with health. But the message then was that fats were bad, while *The Complete Book of Running* by Jim Fixx successfully pitched jogging to the masses. Suddenly, many people associated good health with necessary suffering, because so many enjoyable taste sensations were tarred with the 'bad' brush. Coffee, alcohol, chocolate, olive oil and carbohydrate-heavy foods all, at different times, were relegated to the naughty list, while margarine, low-fat foods and artificial sweeteners seemed like a good idea.

So, what to do, given the conflicting messages that appear to be everywhere? For a start, relax! The 1970s dietary advice that fat was bad had the unforeseen consequence of moving people from high-fat to high-carbohydrate diets, ushering in the modern epidemics of fatty liver disease, diabetes and obesity. But fat isn't bad; indeed a diet high in unsaturated fats has marked health benefits. Jim Fixx, who became a millionaire soon after publishing his guide to running, died of a heart attack during a run at just 52. Science now recognises the potential health consequences of extreme exercise and suggests moderate exercise or high intensity exercise that lasts just seconds may offer the greatest benefits.

Throw off the shackles of kale, boiled cabbage and guilt. Buy a nice bottle of wine, walk to the park and sit in the sun and enjoy a Mediterranean-style meal with friends followed by a café latte.

Chapter 11

To do list – putting liver health on your daily radar

Look after your microbiome

- Avoid antibiotics
- Avoid anti-bacterial sprays
- Get a pet
- Take a probiotic or eat fermented foods:
  - Kimchi
  - Tempeh
  - Yoghurt
  - Kombucha
  - Sauerkraut
  - Miso
- Eat prebiotic foods:
  - Leeks/onions/garlic
  - Jerusalem artichokes
  - Globe artichokes
  - Chicory root
  - Asparagus
  - Bananas (slightly green)
  - Nuts & seeds

Eat

- Choose vegetables and fruit above all else
- Add extra-virgin olive oil liberally to every salad, and fry your food in olive oil as well
- Learn to love lentils, beans, nuts and seeds
- Choose fish, some chicken, and very little red meat
- Avoid anything with added sugar
- Try foods high in resveratrol:
  - Red grapes
  - Peanuts
  - Pistachios
  - Blueberries
  - Cranberries
  - Bilberry
  - Dark chocolate
  - Other grapes
- Include foods containing high levels of anthocyanins:
  - Purple corn
  - Eggplant
  - Blackberries
  - Blueberries
  - Red currants
  - Black currants
  - Blood oranges
  - Cherries
  - Plums
  - Kidney beans
- Add foods high in carotenoids:
  - Sweet potato
  - Carrots
  - Spinach
  - Cos lettuce
  - Butternut squash
  - Cantaloupe
  - Sweet red pepper
  - Dried apricots
  - Peas
  - Broccoli

Indulge

- Enjoy dark chocolate
- Have a daily coffee, or two, or three
- Drink alcohol, but always in moderation!
  - Drink with meals
  - A standard drink contains 10 g of alcohol – no more
  - Moderation for women means up to 2 standard drinks a day, to a total of 7 standard drinks a week
  - Moderation for men means up to 3 standard drinks a day, to a total of 14 standard drinks a week
  - Don't binge drink
  - Understand a hangover means you've gone beyond your body's limit
  - Have between 1 and 4 alcohol-free days every week
  - Drink more water on the days you drink alcohol

Exercise

- Remember, doing nothing for a lot of the day is bad
- Standing and doing nothing is slightly better than sitting and doing nothing
- High intensity, short duration exercise may be as good for you as moderate intensity, moderate duration exercise

Sleep

- Avoid eating or drinking alcohol or coffee after 8 pm most days
- Turn off blue-light devices an hour before bed
- Schedule at least 8 hours of sleep a night
- Get treatment for sleep apnoea

Liver tonics

- Avoid supplementing vitamins A, C & E
- Consider adding turmeric to meals
- Have a salad of bitter greens – maybe even dandelion leaves
- Get adequate sun exposure to boost vitamin D, or take a supplement
- Probiotics actually work – consider taking one

Acknowledgements

I must start by acknowledging my family: Katrina, Nicholas, Oliver, Imogen and Bill. Without their care and support this book would not have been possible. In all of them I see innate wisdom, natural curiosity for the world and an engagement with vulnerability. They make me a slightly better person every day (and there is enormous capacity for improvement).

This book is the distillation of the published papers of hundreds of scientists and doctors. Without their work, this text would not exist and to all of you I am extremely grateful.

I would also like to thank my teachers and colleagues throughout my medical career who have fostered in me an intrinsic enjoyment of medical science and a recognition of the power of evidence-based medicine. I am also indebted to my medical colleagues at the Austin Hospital in Melbourne. Their dedication to patient-centred care and academic excellence is an inspiration to me on a daily basis. Specific recognition also goes to the community of health professionals I work with at the Victorian Liver Transplant Unit – you are a great team.

I would specifically like to thank Kath Knapsey whose role was to wrestle the initial draft of my manuscript into a mature and digestible book. The phrase 'turning a pig's ear into a silk purse' is appropriate for the task Kath undertook. I am also indebted to the team at RMIT and Bowen Street Press; specifically Rose Michael who introduced me to the broader team. Important recognition also goes to Tracy O'Shaughnessy and Cinzia Cavallaro who oversaw the final editing and formatting of the book. Their wisdom, patience and genuine goodwill stood out in every encounter I had with them. Others I want to thank include the student editors at RMIT's Bowen Street Press: Emma Taylor, Natalie Sakarintr, Luke Nichol and Krishna Bhatt. I am also grateful to Phil Campbell for the original cover design, Megan Ellis for text design and layout, and my illustrator Guy Holt.

Finally, I would like to thank the exceptional team at Pan Macmillan Australia, most notably Ingrid Ohlsson, my publisher, and Belinda Huang, my editor.

References

1. N Chalasani, Z Younossi, JE Lavine et al., 'The diagnosis and management of non-alcoholic fatty liver disease: practice guideline by the American Association for the Study of Liver Diseases, American College of Gastroenterology, and the American Gastroenterological Association', *Hepatology*, 2012, 55(6):2005–2023, doi:10.1002/ hep.25762.
2. K Onnerhag, PM Nilsson and S Lindgren, 'Increased risk of cirrhosis and hepatocellular cancer during long-term follow-up of patients with biopsy-proven NAFLD', *Scandinavian Journal of Gastroenterology*, 2014, 49(9):1111–1118, doi:10. 3109/00365521.2014.934911.
3. MB Azad, T Konya, H Maughan et al., 'Infant gut microbiota and the hygiene hypothesis of allergic disease: impact of household pets and siblings on microbiota composition and diversity. Allergy, asthma, and clinical immunology', *Official Journal of the Canadian Society of Allergy and Clinical Immunology*, 2013, 9(1):15, doi:10.1186/1710-1492-9-15.
4. PD Cani, J Amar, MA Iglesias et al., 'Metabolic endotoxemia initiates obesity and insulin resistance', *Diabetes*, 2007, 56(7):1761–1772, doi:10.2337/db06-1491.
5. N Kassaian, A Feizi, A Aminorroaya et al., 'The effects of probiotics and synbiotic supplementation on glucose and insulin metabolism in adults with prediabetes: a double-blind randomized clinical trial', *Acta Diabetologica*, 2018, 55(10):1019– 1028, doi:10.1007/ s00592-018-1175-2.
6. M Ekstedt, H Hagstrom, P Nasr et al., 'Fibrosis stage is the strongest predictor for disease-specific mortality in NAFLD after up to 33 years of follow-up', *Hepatology*, 2015, 61(5):1547–1554, doi:10.1002/hep.27368.
7. C Leung, SW Yeoh, D Patrick et al., 'Characteristics of hepatocellular carcinoma in cirrhotic and non-cirrhotic non-alcoholic fatty liver disease', *World Journal of Gastroenterology*, 2015, 21(4):1189–1196, doi:10.3748/wjg.v21.i4.1189.
8. VW Wong, GL Wong, SW Tsang et al., 'High prevalence of colorectal neoplasm in patients with non-alcoholic steatohepatitis', *Gut*, 2011, 60(6):829–836, doi:1136/gut.2011.239392.
9. C Sanna, C Rosso, M Marietti et al., 'Non-alcoholic fatty liver disease and extra-hepatic cancers', *International Journal of Molecular Sciences*, 2016, 17(5):717, doi:10.3390/ ijms17050717.
10. WD Li, KF Fu, GM Li et al., 'Comparison of effects of obesity and non-alcoholic fatty liver disease on incidence of type 2 diabetes mellitus', *World Journal of Gastroenterology*, 2015, 21(32):9607–9613, doi:10.3748/wjg.v21.i32.9607.
11. The Senate, *Select committee into the obesity epidemic in Australia: final report*, The Senate, Commonwealth of Australia, 2018, accessed 1 January 2019, <http:// www.aph.gov.au/ Parliamentary_Business/Committees/Senate/Obesity_epidemic_ in_Australia/Obesity/Final Report/c01>.
12. Australian Institute of Health and Welfare, *Overweight and obesity in Australia: an updated birth cohort analysis,* Australian Institute of Health and Welfare website, accessed 1 August

2020, <https://www.aihw.gov.au/reports/overweight-obesity/overweight-obesity-updated-birth-cohort-analysis/contents/ background-data-sources-and-methods>.

13. The United States Senate, *Dietary goals for the United States second edition*, Select committee on nutrition and human needs United States Senate, 1977, accessed 1 August 2018, <https://thescienceofnutrition.files.wordpress.com/2014/03/ dietary-goals-for-the-united-states.pdf>.
14. JW Anderson, EC Konz, RC Frederich et al., 'Long-term weight-loss maintenance: a meta-analysis of US studies', *The American Journal of Clinical Nutrition*, 2001, 74(5):579–584, doi:10.1093/ajcn/74.5.579.
15. Deloitte Access Economics, *Economic cost and health burden of liver disease in Australia*, Gastroenterological Society of Australia/Australian Liver Association, 2013.
16. SK Kunutso, TA Apekey, D Seddoh et al., 'Liver enzymes and risk of all-cause mortality in general populations: a systematic review and meta-analysis', *International Journal of Epidemiology*, 2014, 43(1):187–201, doi:10.1093/ije/dyt192.
17. The Lancet, 'Health effects of dietary risks in 195 countries, 1990–2017: a systematic analysis for the Global Burden of Disease Study 2017', *The Lancet*, 2019, doi:10.1016/S0140-6736(19)30041-8.
18. VW Wong, GL Won, AM Chim et al., 'Treatment of nonalcoholic steatohepatitis with probiotics. A proof-of-concept study', *Annals of Hepatology*, 2013, 12(2):256– 262, doi:10.1016/S1665-2681(19)31364-X.
19. N Alang and CR Kelly, 'Weight gain after fecal microbiota transplantation', *Open Forum Infectious Diseases*, 2015, 2(1):ofv004, doi:10.1093/ofid/ofv004.
20. M Dirlewanger, P Schneiter, E Jequier et al., 'Effects of fructose on hepatic glucose metabolism in humans', *American Journal of Physiology. Endocrinology and metabolism*, 2000, 279(4):907–911, doi:10.1152/ajpendo.2000.279.4.E90.
21. KL Stanhope, JM Schwarz, NL Keim et al., 'Consuming fructose-sweetened, not glucose-sweetened, beverages increases visceral adiposity and lipids and decreases insulin sensitivity in overweight/obese humans', *The Journal of Clinical Investigation*, 2009, 119(5):1322–1334, doi:10.112/JCI37385.
22. RD Johnston, MC Stephenson, H Crossland et al., 'No difference between high-fructose and high-glucose diets on liver triacylglycerol or biochemistry in healthy overweight men', *Gastroenterology*, 2013, 145(5):1016–1025, doi:10.1053/j. gastro.2013.07.012.
23. M Maersk, A Belza, H Stodkilde-Jorgensen et al., 'Sucrose-sweetened beverages increase fat storage in the liver, muscle, and visceral fat depot: a 6-mo randomized intervention study', *The American Journal of Clinical Nutrition*, 2012, 95(2):283– 289, doi:10.3945/ajcn.111.022533.
24. JB Schwimmer, P Ugalde-Nicalo, JA Welsh et al., 'Effect of a low free sugar diet vs usual diet on nonalcoholic fatty liver disease in adolescent boys: a randomized clinical trial', *JAMA*, 2019, 321(3):256–265, doi:10.1001/jama.2018.20579.
25. RE Steinert, F Frey, A Topfer et al., 'Effects of carbohydrate sugars and artificial sweeteners on appetite and the secretion of gastrointestinal satiety peptides', *The British Journal of Nutrition*, 105(9):1320–1328, doi:10.1017/ S000711451000512X.
26. N Assy, G Nasser, I Kamayse et al., 'Soft drink consumption linked with fatty liver in the absence of traditional risk factors', *Canadian Journal of Gastroenterology = Journal Canadien de Gastroenterologie*, 2008, 22(10):811–816, doi:10.1155/2008/810961.
27. MF Abdelmalek, A Suzuki, C Guy et al., 'Increased fructose consumption is associated with fibrosis severity in patients with nonalcoholic fatty liver disease', *Hepatology*, 2010, 51(6):1961–1971, doi:10.1002/hep.23535.
28. S Petta, G Marchesini, L Caracausi et al., 'Industrial, not fruit fructose intake is associated with the severity of liver fibrosis in genotype 1 chronic hepatitis C patients', *Journal of Hepatology*, 2013, 59(6):1169–1176, doi:1016/j.jhep.2013.07.037.

29. C Agebratt, E Ström, T Romu et al., 'A Randomized Study of the Effects of Additional Fruit and Nuts Consumption on Hepatic Fat Content, Cardiovascular Risk Factors and Basal Metabolic Rate.' *PLoS ONE*, 2016, 11(1): e0147149. doi.org/10.1371/journal.pone.0147149
30. QP Wang, YQ Lin, L Zhang et al., 'Sucralose promotes food intake through NPY and a neuronal fasting response', *Cell Metabolism*, 2016, 24(1):75–90, doi:10.1016/j. cmet.2016.06.010.
31. J Suez, T Korem, D Zeevi et al., 'Artificial sweeteners induce glucose intolerance by altering the gut microbiota', *Nature*, 2014, 514(7521):181–186, doi:10.1038/ nature13793.
32. Lancet, 'The diet and all-causes death rate in the Seven Countries Study', *Lancet,* 1981, 2(8237):58–6.
33. N Velasco, A Contreras and B Grassi, 'The Mediterranean diet, hepatic steatosis and nonalcoholic fatty liver disease', *Current Opinion in Clinical Nutrition and Metabolic Care,* 2014, 17(5):453–457, doi:10.1097/MCO.0000000000000071.
34. F Turati, D Trichopoulos, J Polesel et al., 'Mediterranean diet and hepatocellular carcinoma', *Journal of Hepatology*, 2014, 60(3):606–611, doi:10.1016/j.jhep.2013.10.034.
35. WQ Li, Y Park, KA McGlynn et al., 'Index-based dietary patterns and risk of incident hepatocellular carcinoma and mortality from chronic liver disease in a prospective study', *Hepatology*, 2014, 60(2):588–597, doi:10.1002/ hep.27160.
36. JF Rinaldi de Alvarenga, P Quifer-Rada, FF Juliano et al., 'Using extra virgin olive oil to cook vegetables enhances polyphenol and carotenoid extractability: a study applying the sofrito technique', *Molecules*, 2019, 24(8):1555, doi:10.3390/ molecules24081555.
37. A Vallverdu-Queralt, J Regueiro, JF Alvarenga et al., 'Carotenoid profile of tomato sauces: effect of cooking time and content of extra virgin olive oil', *International Journal of Molecular Sciences*, 2015, 16(5):9588–9599, doi:10.3390/ijms16059588.
38. JC Kopf, MJ Suhr, J Clarke et al., 'Role of whole grains versus fruits and vegetables in reducing subclinical inflammation and promoting gastrointestinal health in individuals affected by overweight and obesity: a randomized controlled trial', *Journal of Nutrition*, 2018, 1(1):72, doi:10.1186/s12937-018-0381-7.
39. R Chan, VW Wong, WC Chu et al., 'Diet-quality scores and prevalence of nonalcoholic fatty liver disease: a population study using proton-magnetic resonance spectroscopy', *PLoS One*, 2015, 10(9):e0139310, doi:10.1371/journal. pone.0139310.
40. PW Zhang, FX Chen, D Li et al., 'A consort-compliant, randomized, double-blind, placebo-controlled pilot trial of purified anthocyanin in patients with nonalcoholic fatty liver disease', *Medicine,* 2015, 94(20):e758, doi:10.1097/ MD.0000000000000758.
41. NM Wedick, A Pa, A Cassidy et al., 'Dietary flavonoid intakes and risk of type 2 diabetes in US men and women', *The American Journal of Clinical Nutrition*, 2012, 95(4):925–933, doi:10.3945/ajcn.111.028894.
42. B Yilmaz, K Sahin, H Bilen et al., 'Carotenoids and non-alcoholic fatty liver disease', *Hepatobiliary Surgery and Nutrition*, 2015, 4(3):161–171, doi:10.397/j. issn.2304-3881.2015.01.11.
43. DH Lee, MD Gross, DR Jacobs Jr, 'Association of serum carotenoids and tocopherols with gamma-glutamyltransferase: the Cardiovascular Risk Development in Young Adults (CARDIA) Study', *Clinical Chemistry*, 2004, 50(3):582–588, doi:10.1373/ clinchem.2003.028852.
44. J Liu, WQ Shi, Y Cao et al., 'Higher serum carotenoid concentrations associated with a lower prevalence of the metabolic syndrome in middle-aged and elderly Chinese adults', *The British Journal of Nutrition*, 2014, 112(12):2041–2048, doi:10.1017/ S000711451400316X.
45. S Zhang, J Fu, Q Zhang et al., 'Association between nut consumption and non-alcoholic fatty liver disease in adults', *Liver International*, 2019, 39(9):1732–1741, doi:10.1111/liv.14164.

46. R Cueto-Galan, FJ Baron, P Valdivielso et al., 'Changes in fatty liver index after consuming a Mediterranean diet: 6-year follow-up of the PREDIMED-Malaga trial', *Medicina Clinica*, 2016, 148(10), doi:10.1016/j.medcle.2017.04.030.
47. SB Eaton, SB Eaton 3rd, MJ Konner et al., 'An evolutionary perspective enhances understanding of human nutritional requirements', *Journal of Nutrition*, 1996, 126(6):132–40, doi:10.1093/jn/126.6.1732.
48. F Fayet-Moore, T Cassettari, K Tuck et al., 'Dietary fibre intake in Australia. Paper I: associations with demographic, socio-economic, and anthropometric factors', *Nutrients*, 2018, 10(5):599, doi:10.3390/nu10050599.
49. G Musso, R Gambino, F De Michieli et al., 'Dietary habits and their relations to insulin resistance and postprandial lipemia in nonalcoholic steatohepatitis', *Hepatology*, 2003, 37(4):909–916, doi:10.1053/jhep.2003.50132.
50. Y Cheng, K Zhang, Y Chen et al., 'Associations between dietary nutrient intakes and hepatic lipid contents in NAFLD patients quantified by (1)H-MRS and dual-echo MRI', *Nutrients*, 2016, 8(9):527, doi:10.3390/nu8090527.
51. CA Daubioul, Y Horsmans, P Lambert et al., 'Effects of oligofructose on glucose and lipid metabolism in patients with nonalcoholic steatohepatitis: results of a pilot study', *European Journal of Clinical Nutrition*, 2005, 59(5):23–26, doi:10.1038/ sj.ejcn.1602127.
52. M Krawczyk, D Maciejewska, K Ryterska et al., 'Gut permeability might be improved by dietary fiber in individuals with nonalcoholic fatty liver disease (NAFLD) undergoing weight reduction', *Nutrients*, 2018, 10(11):1793, doi:10.3390/nu10111793.
53. V Fedirko, A Trichopolou, C Bamia et al., 'Consumption of fish and meats and risk of hepatocellular carcinoma: the European Prospective Investigation into Cancer and Nutrition (EPIC)', *Annals of Oncology: Official Journal of the European Society for Medical Oncology*, 2013, 24(8):2166–2173, doi:10.1093/annonc/mdt168.
54. J Luo, Y Yang, J Liu et al., 'Systematic review with meta-analysis: meat consumption and the risk of hepatocellular carcinoma', *Alimentary Pharmacology & Therapeutics*, 2014, 39(9): 913–922, doi:10.1111/apt.12678.
55. ND Freedman, AJ Cross, KA McGlynn et al., 'Association of meat and fat intake with liver disease and hepatocellular carcinoma in the NIH-AARP cohort', *Journal of the National Cancer Institute*, 2010, 102(17):1354–1365, doi:10.1093/jnci/djq301.
56. M Georgoulis, MD Kontogianni, A Margariti et al., 'Associations between dietary intake and the presence of the metabolic syndrome in patients with non-alcoholic fatty liver disease', *Journal of Human Nutrition and Dietetics: The Official Journal of the British Dietetic Association*, 2015, 28(4):409–415, doi:10.1111/jhn.12323.
57. S Zelber-Sagi, D Ivancovsky-Wajcman, NF Isakov et al., 'High red and processed meat consumption is associated with non-alcoholic fatty liver disease and insulin resistance', *Journal of Hepatology*, 2018, 68(6):1239–1246, doi:10.1016/j. jhep.2018.01.015.
58. LJ Rogers, AG Basnakian, MS Orloff et al., '2-amino-1-methyl-6-phenylimidazo (4,5-b) pyridine (PhIP) induces gene expression changes in JAK/STAT and MAPK pathways related to inflammation, diabetes and cancer', *Nutrition and Metabolism*, 2016, 13:54, doi:10.1186/s12986-016-0111-0.
59. PK Luukkonen, S Sadevirta, Y Zhou et al., 'Saturated fat is more metabolically harmful for the human liver than unsaturated fat or simple sugars', *Diabetes Care*, 2018, 41(8):dc 180071, doi:10.2337/dc18-0071.
60. L Eyres, MF Eyres, A Chisholm et al., 'Coconut oil consumption and cardiovascular risk factors in humans', *Nutrition Reviews*, 2016, 74(4):267–80, doi:10.1093/nutrit/nuw002.
61. P Nigam, S Bhatt, A Misra et al., 'Effect of a 6-month intervention with cooking oils containing a high concentration of monounsaturated fatty acids (olive and canola oils)

compared with control oil in male Asian Indians with nonalcoholic fatty liver disease', *Diabetes Technology & Therapeutics*, 2014, 16(4):255–261, doi:10.1089/dia.2013.0178.
62. YH Li, LH Yang, KH Sha et al., 'Efficacy of poly-unsaturated fatty acid therapy on patients with nonalcoholic steatohepatitis', *World Journal of Gastroenterology*, 2015, 21(22):7008–7013, doi:10.3748/wjf.v21.i22.7008.
63. T Duarte-Salles, V Fedirko, M Stepien et al., 'Dietary fat, fat subtypes and hepatocellular carcinoma in a large European cohort', *International Journal of Cancer*, 2015, 137(11):2715–2728, doi:10.1002/ijc.29643.
64. T Duarte-Salles, V Fedirko, M Stepien et al., 'Dairy products and risk of hepatocellular carcinoma: the European prospective investigation into cancer and nutrition', *International Journal of Cancer*, 2014, 135(7):1662–1672, doi:10.1002/ijc.28812.
65. CE Dugan, D Aguilar, YK Park et al., 'Dairy consumption lowers systemic inflammation and liver enzymes in typically low-dairy consumers with clinical characteristics of metabolic syndrome', *Journal of the American College of Nutrition*, 2016, 35(3):255–261, doi:10.1080/07315724.2015.1022637.
66. F Bakhshimoghaddam, K Shateri, M Sina et al., 'Daily consumption of synbiotic yogurt decreases liver steatosis in patients with nonalcoholic fatty liver disease: a randomized controlled clinical trial', *The Journal of Nutrition*, 2018, 148(8): 1541–6100, doi:10.1093/jn/nxy088.
67. S Nabavi, M Rafraf, MH Somi et al., 'Effects of probiotic yogurt consumption on metabolic factors in individuals with nonalcoholic fatty liver disease', *Journal of Dairy Science*, 2014, 97(12):7386–7393, doi:10.2168/jds.2013-8500.
68. A Alkerwi, N Sauvageot, G Crichton et al., 'Daily chocolate consumption is inversely associated with insulin resistance and liver enzymes in the Observation of Cardiovascular Risk Factors in Luxembourg Study', *British Journal of Nutrition*, 115(9):1475–2662, doi:10.1017/S0007114516000702.
69. I Rodriguez-Ramiro, D Vauzour and AM Minihane, 'Polyphenols and non-alcoholic fatty liver disease: impact and mechanisms', *The Proceedings of the Nutrition Society*, 2016, 75(1): 47–60, doi:10.1017/S0029665115004218.
70. A Moreira, MJ Diogenes, A de Mendonca et al., 'Chocolate consumption is associated with a lower risk of cognitive decline', *Journal of Alzheimer's Disease*, 2016, 53(1):85–93, doi:10.3233/JAD-160142.
71. G Desideri, C Kwik-Uribe, D Grassi et al., 'Benefits in cognitive function, blood pressure, and insulin resistance through cocoa flavanol consumption in elderly subjects with mild cognitive impairment: the Cocoa, Cognition, and Aging (CoCoA) Study', *Hypertension*, 2012, 60(3):794–801, doi:10.1161/ HYPERTENSIONAHA.112.193060.
72. D Mastroiacovo, C Kwik-Uribe, D Grassi et al., 'Cocoa flavanol consumption improves cognitive function, blood pressure control, and metabolic profile in elderly subjects: the Cocoa, Cognition, and Aging (CoCoA) Study – a randomized controlled trial', *The American Journal of Clinical Nutrition*, 2015, 101(3):538–548, doi:10.3945/ajcn.114.092189.
73. LA Massee, K Ried, M Pase et al., 'The acute and sub-chronic effects of cocoa flavanols on mood, cognitive and cardiovascular health in young healthy adults: a randomized, controlled trial', *Frontiers in Pharmacology*, 2015, 6(93), doi:10.3389/ fphar.2015.00093.
74. DT Field, CM Williams and LT Butler, 'Consumption of cocoa flavanols results in an acute improvement in visual and cognitive functions', *Physiology & Behavior*, 2011, 103(3–4): 255–260, doi:10.1016/j.physbeh.2011.02.013.
75. AN Sokolov, MA Pavlova, S Klosterhalfen et al., 'Chocolate and the brain: neurobiological impact of cocoa flavanols on cognition and behavior', *Neuroscience and Biobehavioral Reviews*, 2013, 37(10 Pt 2):2445–2453, doi:10.1016/j. neubiorev.2013.06.013.
76. FH Messerli, 'Chocolate consumption, cognitive function, and Nobel Laureates', *The New England Journal of Medicine*, 2012, 367(16):1562–1564, doi:10.1056/ NEJMon1211064.

77. Forbes, 'The world's biggest chocolate consumers 2015', *Forbes*, 22 July 2015, accessed 1 August 2018, <http://www.forbes.com/sites/niallmccarthy/2015/07/22/ the-worlds-biggest-chocolate-consumers-infographic/>.
78. M Weisenberg, Y Gerby and M Mikulincer, 'Aerobic exercise and chocolate as means for reducing learned helplessness', *Cognitive Therapy and Research*, 1993, 17(6):579–592, doi:10.1007/BF01176080.
79. NK Hollenberg, G Martinez, M McCullough et al., 'Aging, acculturation, salt intake, and hypertension in the Kuna of Panama', *Hypertension*, 1997, 29(1 Pt 2):171–176, doi:10.1161/01.hyp.29.1.171.
80. V Bayard, F Chamorro, J Motta et al., 'Does flavanol intake influence mortality from nitric oxide-dependent processes? Ischemic heart disease, stroke, diabetes mellitus, and cancer in Panama', *International Journal of Medical Sciences*, 2007, 4(1):53–58, doi:10.7150/ijms.4.53.
81. B Buijsse, EJM Feskens, FJ Kok et al., 'Cocoa intake, blood pressure, and cardiovascular mortality: the Zutphen Elderly Study', *Archives of Internal Medicine*, 2006, 166(4):411–417, doi:101001/archinte.166.4.411.
82. M Cuenca-Garcia, JR Ruiz, FB Ortega et al., 'Association between chocolate consumption and fatness in European adolescents', *Nutrition*, 2014, 30(2):236–239, doi:10.1016/j.nut.2013.07.011.
83. JA Greenberg and B Buijsse, 'Habitual chocolate consumption may increase body weight in a dose-response manner', *PloS ONE*, 2013, 8(8):e70271, doi:10.1371/ journal.pone.0070271.
84. G Farhat, S Drummond, L Fyfe et al., 'Dark chocolate: an obesity paradox or a culprit for weight gain?', *Phytotherapy Research*, 2014, 28(6):791–797, doi:10.1002/ ptr.5062.
85. ML Chen, L Yi, Y Zhang et al., 'Resveratrol attenuates Trimethylamine-N-Oxide (TMAO)-induced atherosclerosis by regulating TMAO synthesis and bile acid metabolism via remodeling of the gut microbiota', *mBio*, 2016, 7(2):e02210–02215, doi:10.1128/mBio.02210-15.
86. F Faghihzadeh, P Adibi and A Hekmatdoost, 'The effects of resveratrol supplementation on cardiovascular risk factors in patients with non-alcoholic fatty liver disease: a randomised, double-blind, placebo-controlled study', *The British Journal of Nutrition*, 2015, 114(5): 796–803, doi:10.1017/s0007114515002433.
87. K Kantartzis, L Fritsche, M Bombrich et al., 'Effects of resveratrol supplementation on liver fat content in overweight and insulin-resistant subjects: a randomized, double-blind, placebo-controlled clinical trial', *Diabetes, Obesity and Metabolism*, 2018, 20(7):1793–1797, doi:10.1111/dom.13268.
88. DG Schlundt, JO Hill, T Sbrocco et al., 'The role of breakfast in the treatment of obesity: a randomized clinical trial', *The American Journal of Clinical Nutrition*, 1992, 55(3):645–651, doi:10.1093/ajcn/55.3.645.
89. RI Versteeg, MT Ackermans, AJ Nederveen et al., 'Meal timing effects on insulin sensitivity and intrahepatic triglycerides during weight loss', *International Journal of Obesity*, 2018, 42(2):156–162, doi:10.1038/ijo.2017.199.
90. T Nishi, A Babazono, T Maeda et al., 'Effects of eating fast and eating before bedtime on the development of nonalcoholic fatty liver disease', *Population Health Management*, 2016, 19(4):279–283, doi:10.1089/pop.2015.0088.
91. RE Patterson and DD Sears, 'Metabolic effects of intermittent fasting', *Annual Review of Nutrition*, 2017, 37:371–393, doi:10.1146/annurev-nutr-071816-064634.
92. KE Koopman, MWA Caan, AJ Nederveen et al., 'Hypercaloric diets with increased meal frequency, but not meal size, increase intrahepatic triglycerides: a randomized controlled trial', *Hepatology*, 2014, 60(2):545–553, doi:10.1002/hep.27149.
93. JF Trepanowski, CM Kroeger, A Barnosky et al., 'Effect of alternate-day fasting on weight loss, weight maintenance, and cardioprotection among metabolically healthy obese adults:

a randomized clinical trial', *JAMA Internal Medicine*, 2017, 177(7):930–938, doi:10.1001/jamainternmed.2017.0936.

94. F Aliasghari, A Izadi, BP Gargari et al., 'The effects of ramadan fasting on body composition, blood pressure, glucose metabolism, and markers of inflammation in NAFLD patients: an observational trial', *Journal of the American College of Nutrition*, 2017, 36(8):640–645, doi:10.1 080/07315724.2017.1339644.
95. S Ponte, 'The "latte revolution"? Regulation, markets and consumption in the global coffee chain', *World Development*, 2002, 30(7):1099–1122, doi:10.1016/ S0305-750X(02)00032-3.
96. K Bernard, *Top 10 coffee consuming nations*, WorldAtlas, 2020, accessed 1 August 2018, <http://www.worldatlas.com/articles/top-10-coffee-consuming-nations. html>.
97. J Foster, 'Caffeine (coffee) consumption by country', *Caffeine Informer*, 15 October 2018, accessed 1 August 2019, <http://www.caffeineinformer.com/ caffeine-what-the-world-drinks>.
98. MJ Couvillon, HA Toufailia, TM Butterfield et al., 'Caffeinated forage tricks honeybees into increasing foraging and recruitment behaviors', *Current Biology*, 2015, 25(21):2815–2818, doi:10.1016/j.cub.2015.08.052.
99. MC Cornelis and A El-Sohemy, 'Coffee, caffeine, and coronary heart disease', *Current Opinion in Clinical Nutrition & Metabolic Care*, 2007, 10(6):745–751, doi:10.1097/MCO.0b013e328f05d81.
100. E Arnesen, NE Huseby, T Brenn et al., 'The Tromsø Heart Study: distribution of, and determinants for, gamma-glutamyltransferase in a free-living population', *Scandinavian Journal of Clinical and Laboratory Investigation*, 1986, 46(1):63–70, doi:10.3109/0036551 8609086483.
101. O Nilssen, OH Forde and T Brenn, 'The Tromsø Study. Distribution and population determinants of gamma-glutamyltransferase', *American Journal of Epidemiology*, 1990, 132(2):318–326, doi:10.1093/oxfordjournals.aje.a115661.
102. E Casiglia, P Spolaore, G Ginocchio et al., 'Unexpected effects of coffee consumption on liver enzymes', *European Journal of Epidemiology*, 1993, 9(3):293– 297, doi:10.1007/bf00146266.
103. Q Xiao, R Sinha, BI Graubard et al., 'Inverse associations of total and decaffeinated coffee with liver enzyme levels in National Health and Nutrition Examination Survey 1999–2010', *Hepatology*, 2014, 60(6):2091–2098, doi:10.1002/hep.27367.
104. A Hodge, S Lim, E Goh et al., 'Coffee intake is associated with a lower liver stiffness in patients with non-alcoholic fatty liver disease, hepatitis C, and hepatitis B', *Nutrients*, 2017, 9(1):2072–6643, doi:10.3390/nu9010056.
105. K Friedrich, M Smit, A Wannhoff et al., 'Coffee consumption protects against progression in liver cirrhosis and increases long-term survival after liver transplantation', *Journal of Gastroenterology and Hepatology*, 2016, 31(8):1470–1475, doi:10.1111/jgh.13319.
106. S Zelber-Sagi, F Salomone, M Webb et al., 'Coffee consumption and nonalcoholic fatty liver onset: a prospective study in the general population', *Translational Research*, 2015, 165(3):428–436, doi:10.1016/j.trsl.2014.10.008.
107. JW Molloy, CJ Calcagno, CD Williams et al., 'Association of coffee and caffeine consumption with fatty liver disease, nonalcoholic steatohepatitis, and degree of hepatic fibrosis', *Hepatology*, 2012, 55(2):429–436, doi:10.1002/help.24731.
108. G Corrao, A Zambon, V Bagnardi et al., 'Coffee, caffeine, and the risk of liver cirrhosis', *Annals of Epidemiology*, 2001, 11(7):458–465, doi:10.1016/ s1047-2797(01)00223-x.
109. VW Setiawan, LR Wilkens, SC Lu et al., 'Association of coffee intake with reduced incidence of liver cancer and death from chronic liver disease in the US multiethnic cohort', *Gastroenterology*, 2015, 148(1):118–125, doi:10,1053/j. gastro.2014.10.005.

110. A Jemal, F Bray, J Ferlay et al., 'Global cancer statistics', *CA: A Cancer Journal for Clinicians*, 2011, 61(2):69–90, doi:10.3322/caac.20107.
111. K Tanaka, M Hara, T Sakamoto et al., 'Inverse association between coffee drinking and the risk of hepatocellular carcinoma: a case-control study in Japan', *Cancer Science*, 2007, 98(2):214–218, doi:10.1111/j.1349-7006.2006.00368.x.
112. WW Leung, SC Ho, HL Chan et al., 'Moderate coffee consumption reduces the risk of hepatocellular carcinoma in hepatitis B chronic carriers: a case-control study', *Journal of Epidemiology and Community Health*, 2011, 65(6):556–558, doi:10.1136/jech.2009.104125.
113. M Montella, J Polesel, C La Vecchia et al., 'Coffee and tea consumption and risk of hepatocellular carcinoma in Italy', *International Journal of Cancer*, 2007, 120(7):1555–1559, doi:10.1002/ijc.22509.
114. GB Goh, WC Chow, JM Yuan et al., 'Coffee, alcohol and other beverages in relation to cirrhosis mortality: the Singapore Chinese Health Study', *Hepatology*, 2014, 60(2):661–669, doi:10.1002/hep.27054.
115. JH Hankin, DO Stram, K Arakawa et al., 'Singapore Chinese Health Study: development, validation, and calibration of the quantitative food frequency questionnaire', *Nutrition and Cancer*, 39(2):187–195, doi:10.1207/S15327914nc392_5.
116. M Noordzij, CS Uiterwaal, LR Arends et al., 'Blood pressure response to chronic intake of coffee and caffeine: a meta-analysis of randomized controlled trials', *Journal of Hypertension*, 2005, 23(5):921–928, doi:10.1097/01. hjh.0000166828.94699.1d..
117. I Tanida, Y Shirasago, R Suzuki et al., 'Inhibitory effects of caffeic acid, a coffee-related organic acid, on the propagation of hepatitis C virus', *Japanese Journal of Infectious Diseases*, 2015, 68(4):268–275, doi:10.7883/yoken.JJID.2014.309.
118. V Lecoultre, G Carrel, L Egli et al., 'Coffee consumption attenuates short-term fructose-induced liver insulin resistance in healthy men', *The American Journal of Clinical Nutrition*, 2014, 99(2):268–275, doi:10.3945/ajcn.113.069526.
119. CE Mills, X Tzounis, MJ Oruna-Concha et al., 'In vitro colonic metabolism of coffee and chlorogenic acid results in selective changes in human faecal microbiota growth', *British Journal of Nutrition*, 2015, 113(8):1220–1227, doi:10.1017/ S0007114514003948.
120. K Velickovic, D Wayne, HAL Leija et al., 'Caffeine exposure induces browning features in adipose tissue in vitro and in vivo', *Scientific Reports*, 2019, 9(1):9104, doi:10.1038/s41598-019-45540-1.
121. M Steffen, C Kuhle, D Hensrud et al., 'The effect of coffee consumption on blood pressure and the development of hypertension: a systematic review and meta-analysis', *Journal of Hypertension*, 2012, 30(12):2245–2254, doi:10.1097/ HJH.0b012e3283588d73.
122. I Guessous, CB Eap and M Bochud, 'Blood pressure in relation to coffee and caffeine consumption', *Current Hypertension Reports*, 2014, 16(9):468, doi:10.1007/ s11906-014-0468-2.
123. R Huxley, CM Lee, F Barzi et al., 'Coffee, decaffeinated coffee, and tea consumption in relation to incident type 2 diabetes mellitus: a systematic review with meta-analysis', *Archives of Internal Medicine*, 2009, 169(22):2053–2063, doi:10.1001/archinternmed.2009.439.
124. T Bahorun, A Luximon-Ramma, VS Neergheen-Bhujun et al., 'The effect of black tea on risk factors of cardiovascular disease in a normal population', *Preventive Medicine*, 2012, (54) Suppl:S98–102, doi:10.1016/j.ypmed.2011.12.009.
125. G Grosso, U Stepaniak, A Micek et al., 'Coffee consumption and mortality in three Eastern European countries: results from the HAPIEE (Health, Alcohol and Psychosocial factors In Eastern Europe) study', *Public Health Nutrition*, 2017, 20(1):82–91, doi:10.1017/ S1368980016001749.
126. JH O'Keefe, SK Bhatti, HR Patil et al., 'Effects of habitual coffee consumption on cardiometabolic disease, cardiovascular health, and all-cause mortality', *Journal of the American College of Cardiology*, 2013, 62(12):1043–1051, doi:10.1016/j. jacc.2013.06.035.

127. ND Freedman, Y Park, CC Abnet et al., 'Association of coffee drinking with total and cause-specific mortality', *The New England Journal of Medicine*, 2012, 366(20):1891–1904, doi:10.1056/NEJMoa1112010.
128. H Liu, K Yao, W Zhang et al., 'Coffee consumption and risk of fractures: a meta-analysis', *Archives of Medical Science*, 2012, 8(5):776–783, doi:10.5114/ aoms.2012.31612.
129. ME Mattson, 'Update on emergency department visits involving energy drinks: a continuing public health concern', *The CBHSQ Report, Rockville (MD): Substance Abuse and Mental Health Services Administration (US)*, 2013.
130. N Gunja and JA Brown, 'Energy drinks: health risks and toxicity', *The Medical Journal of Australia*, 2012, 196(1):46–49, doi:10.5694/mja11.10838.
131. S Avci, R Sarikaya and F Buyukcam, 'Death of a young man after overuse of energy drink', *The American Journal of Emergency Medicine*, 2013, 31(11):1624. e1623–1624, doi:10.1016/j. ajem.2013.06.031.
132. SB Jabbar and MG Hanly, 'Fatal caffeine overdose: a case report and review of literature', *The American Journal of Forensic Medicine and Pathology*, 2013, 34(4):321–324, doi:10.1097/ PAF.0000000000000058.
133. LE Armstrong, DJ Casa, CM Maresh et al., 'Caffeine, fluid-electrolyte balance, temperature regulation, and exercise-heat tolerance', *Exercise and Sport Sciences Reviews*, 2007, 35(3): 135-140, doi:10.1097/jes.0b013e3180a02cc1.
134. RD Deegan, 'Capillary flow as the cause of ring stains from dried liquid drops', *Nature*, 1997, 389:827–829, doi:10.1038/39827.
135. MA Carrigan, O Uryasev, CB Frye et al., 'Hominids adapted to metabolize ethanol long before human-directed fermentation', *Proceedings of the National Academy of Sciences*, 2014, 112(2):1091–6490, doi:10.1073/pnas.1404167111.
136. M Chuhrova and I Timofeyev, 'Synthesis of endogenous ethanol during treatment of alcoholic dependence', *European Psychiatry*, 2012, (17)Suppl1:191, doi:10.1016/ S0924-9338(02)80818-5.
137. RG Ladkin and JN Davies, 'Rupture of the stomach in an African child', *British Medical Journal*, 1948, 1(4552):644, doi:10.1136/bmj.1.4552.644.
138. BK Logan and AW Jones, 'Endogenous ethanol "auto-brewery syndrome" as a drunk-driving defence challenge', *Medicine, Science, and the Law*, 2000, 40(3):206–215, doi:10.1177/002580240004000304.
139. A Dahshan and K Donovan, 'Auto-brewery syndrome in a child with short gut syndrome: case report and review of the literature', *Journal of Pediatric Gastroenterology and Nutrition*, 2001, 33(2):214–215, doi:10.1097/00005176-200108000-00024.
140. SR Gochman, MB Brown and NJ Dominy, 'Alcohol discrimination and preferences in two species of nectar-feeding primate', *Royal Society Open Science*, 2016, 3(7):160217, doi:10.1098/rsos.160217.
141. KJ Hockings, N Bryson-Morrison, S Carvalho et al., 'Tools to tipple: ethanol ingestion by wild chimpanzees using leaf-sponges', *Royal Society Open Science*, 2015, 2(6):150150, doi:10.1098/rsos.150150.
142. AI Cederbaum, 'Alcohol metabolism', *Clinics in Liver Disease*, 2012, 16(4):667–685, doi:10.1016/j.cld.2012.08.002.
143. U Becker, M Gronbaek, D Johansen et al., 'Lower risk for alcohol-induced cirrhosis in wine drinkers', *Hepatology*, 2002, 35(4):868–875, doi:10.1053/jhep.2002.32101.
144. W Dunn, AJ Sanyal, EM Brunt et al., 'Modest alcohol consumption is associated with decreased prevalence of steatohepatitis in patients with non-alcoholic fatty liver disease (NAFLD)', *Journal of Hepatology*, 2012, 57(2):384–391, doi:10.1016/j. jhep.2012.03.024.

145. W Dunn, R Xu and JB Schwimmer, 'Modest wine drinking and decreased prevalence of suspected nonalcoholic fatty liver disease', *Hepatology*, 2008, 47(6):1947–1954, doi:10.1002/hep.22292.
146. MM Joosten, JW Beulens, S Kersten et al., 'Moderate alcohol consumption increases insulin sensitivity and ADIPOQ expression in postmenopausal women: a randomised, crossover trial', *Diabetologica*, 2008, 51(8):1375–81, doi:10.1007/ s00125-008-1031-y.
147. PV Kenkre, RD Lindeman, CL Yau et al., 'Serum insulin concentrations in daily drinkers compared with abstainers in the New Mexico elder health survey', *The Journals of Gerontology: Series A,* 2003, 58(10):M960–963, doi:10.1093/gerona/58.10.M960.
148. JB Dixon, PS Bhathal and PE O'Brien, 'Nonalcoholic fatty liver disease: predictors of nonalcoholic steatohepatitis and liver fibrosis in the severely obese', *Gastroenterology*, 2001, 121(1):91–100, doi:10.1053/gast.2001.25540.
149. PE Ronksley, SE Brien, BJ Turner et al., 'Association of alcohol consumption with selected cardiovascular disease outcomes: a systematic review and meta-analysis', *BMJ*, 2011, 342:d671, doi:10.1136/bmj.d671.
150. R Vliegenthart, HS Oei, A Van den Elzen et al., 'Alcohol consumption and coronary calcification in a general population', *Archives of Internal Medicine*, 2004, 164(21):2355–60, doi:10.1001/archinte.164.21.2355.
151. MJ Davies, DJ Baer, JT Judd et al., 'Effects of moderate alcohol intake on fasting insulin and glucose concentrations and insulin sensitivity in postmenopausal women: a randomized controlled trial', *Journal of the American Medical Association*, 2002, 287(19):2559–2562, doi:10.1001/jama.287.19.2559.
152. A Sierksma, H Patel, N Ouchi et al., 'Effect of moderate alcohol consumption on adiponectin, tumor necrosis factor-alpha, and insulin sensitivity', *Diabetes Care*, 2004, 27(1):184–189, doi:10.2337/diacare.27.1.184.
153. LL Koppes, JM Dekker, HF Hendriks et al., 'Moderate alcohol consumption lowers the risk of type 2 diabetes: a meta-analysis of prospective observational studies', *Diabetes Care*, 2005, 28(3):719–725, doi:10.2337/diacare.28.3.719.
154. C Bate and A Williams, 'Ethanol protects cultured neurons against amyloid-beta and alpha-synuclein-induced synapse damage', *Neuropharmacology*, 2011, 61(8):1406–1412, doi:10.1016/j.neuropharm.2011.08.030.
155. JH O'Keefe, KA Bybee and CJ Lavie, 'Alcohol and cardiovascular health: the razor-sharp double-edged sword', *Journal of the American College of Cardiology*, 2007, 50(11):1009–1014, doi:10.1016/j.jacc.2007.04.089.
156. MS Elkind, R Sciacca, B Boden-Albala et al., 'Moderate alcohol consumption reduces risk of ischemic stroke: the Northern Manhattan Study', *Stroke*, 2006, 31(1):13–19, doi:10.1161/01.STR.0000195048.86810.5b.
157. A Poli, F Marangoni, A Avogaro et al., 'Moderate alcohol use and health: a consensus document', *Nutrition, Metabolism, and Cardiovascular Diseases*, 2013, 23(6):487–504, doi:10.1016/j.numecd.2013.02.007.
158. MB Wozniak, P Brennan, DR Brenner et al., 'Alcohol consumption and the risk of renal cancers in the European prospective investigation into cancer and nutrition (EPIC)', *International Journal of Cancer*, 2015, 137(8):1953–1966, doi:10.1002/ ijc.29559.
159. NE Allen, V Beral, D Casabonne et al., 'Moderate alcohol intake and cancer incidence in women', *Journal of the National Cancer Institute*, 2009, 101(5):296–305, doi:10.1093/jnci/djn514.
160. P Boyle and P Boffetta, 'Alcohol consumption and breast cancer risk', *Breast Cancer Research: BCR*, 2009, 11(Suppl 3):S3, doi:10.1186/bcr2422.
161. MG O'Doherty, K Cairns, V O'Neill, et al., 'Effect of major lifestyle risk factors, independent and jointly, on life expectancy with and without cardiovascular disease: results

from the Consortium on Health and Ageing Network of Cohorts in Europe and the United States (CHANCES)', *European Journal of Epidemiology*, 2016, 31(5):455–468, doi:10.1007/s10654-015-0112-8.

162. G Farchi, F Fidanza, S Giampaoli et al., 'Alcohol and survival in the Italian rural cohorts of the Seven Countries Study', *International Journal of Epidemiology*, 2000, 29(4):667–671, doi:10.1093/ije/29.4.667.
163. Y Gepner, R Golan, I Harman-Boehm et al., 'Effects of initiating moderate alcohol intake on cardiometabolic risk in adults with type 2 diabetes: a 2-year randomized, controlled trial', *Annals of Internal Medicine*, 2015, 163(8):569–579, doi:10.7326/M14-1650.
164. C Sayon-Orea, MA Martinez-Gonzalez and M Bes-Rastrollo, 'Alcohol consumption and body weight: a systematic review', *Nutrition Reviews,* 2011, 69(8):419–31, doi:10.1111/j.1753-4887.2011.00403.x.
165. Y Gepner, Y Henkin, D Schwarzfuchs et al., 'Differential effect of initiating moderate red wine consumption on 24-h blood pressure by alcohol dehydrogenase genotypes: randomized trial in type 2 diabetes', *American Journal of Hypertension*, 2016, 29(4):476–483, doi:10.1093/ajh/hpv126.
166. MA Noguer, AB Cerezo, ED Navarro et al., 'Intake of alcohol-free red wine modulates antioxidant enzyme activities in a human intervention study', *Pharmacological Research*, 2012, 65(6):609–614, doi:10.1016/j.phrs.2012.03.003.
167. S Arranz, G Chiva-Blanch, P Valderas-Martinez et al., 'Wine, beer, alcohol and polyphenols on cardiovascular disease and cancer', *Nutrients*, 2012, 4(7):759–781, doi:10.3390/nu4070759.
168. KA McCaul, OP Almeida, GJ Hankey et al., 'Alcohol use and mortality in older men and women', *Addiction*, 2010, 105(8):1391–1400, doi:10.1111/ j.1360-0443.2010.02972.x
169. KJ Mukamal, M Maclure, JE Muller et al., 'Binge drinking and mortality after acute myocardial infarction', *Circulation*, 2005, 112(25):3839–3845, doi:10.1161/CIRCULATIONAHA.105.574749.
170. R Swift and D Davidson, 'Alcohol hangover: Mechanisms and mediators', *Alcohol Health and Research World*, 1998, 22(1):54–60.
171. OK Vartia, OA Forsander and FE Krusius, 'Blood sugar values in hangover', *Quarterly Journal of Studies on Alcohol*, 1960, 21(4):579–604, doi:10.15288/qjsa.1960.21.597.
172. M Takahashi, W Li, K Koike et al., 'Clinical effectiveness of KSS formula, a traditional folk remedy for alcohol hangover symptoms', *Journal of Natural Medicines*, 2010, 64(4):487–491, doi:10.1007/s11418-010-0430-9.
173. GL Pawan, 'Alcoholic drinks and hangover effects', *The Proceedings of the Nutrition Society*, 1973, 32(1):15a.
174. JC Verster and R Penning, 'Treatment and prevention of alcohol hangover', *Current Drug Abuse Reviews*, 2010, 3(2):103–109, doi:10.2174/1874473711003020 103.
175. M Trevisan, E Schisterman, A Mennotti et al., 'Drinking pattern and mortality: the Italian Risk Factor and Life Expectancy pooling project', *Annals of Epidemiology*, 2001, 11(5): 312–319, doi:10.1016/S1047-2797(00)00183-6.
176. S Stranges, T Wu, JM Dorn et al., 'Relationship of alcohol drinking pattern to risk of hypertension: a population-based study', *Hypertension*, 2004, 44(6):813–819, doi:10.1161/01.HYP.0000146537.03103.f2.
177. M Boban, C Stockley, PL Teissedre et al., 'Drinking pattern of wine and effects on human health: why should we drink moderately and with meals?', *Food & Function*, 2016, 7(7): 2937–2942, doi:10.1039/C6FO00218H.
178. CA Burton, *Alcohol consumption by country*, WorldAtlas, 2018, accessed 1 August 2019, <http://www.worldatlas.com/articles/who-drinks-the-most-alcohol-consumption-by-country.html>.

179. R Pechey, DL Couturier, GJ Hollands et al., 'Does wine glass size influence sales for on-site consumption? A multiple treatment reversal design', *BMC Public Health*, 2016, 16:390, doi:10.1186/s12889-016-3068-z.
180. KM Keyes, E Calvo, KA Ornstein et al., 'Alcohol consumption in later life and mortality in the United States: results from 9 waves of the Health and Retirement Study', *Alcohol Clinical and Experimental Research*, 2019, 43(8):1734–1746, doi:10.1111/acer.14125.
181. DM von Conrady and A Bonney, 'Patterns of complementary and alternative medicine use and health literacy in general practice patients in urban and regional Australia', *Australian Family Physician*, 2017, 46(5):316–320.
182. CCL Xue, AL Zhang, V Lin et al., 'Complementary and alternative medicine use in Australia: a national population-based survey', *The Journal of Alternative and Complementary Medicine*, 2007, 13(6):643–650, doi:10.1089/acm.2006.6355.
183. A Rambaldi, BP Jacobs and C Gluud, 'Milk thistle for alcoholic and/or hepatitis B or C virus liver diseases', *Cochrane Database of Systematic Reviews*, 2007, (4):CD003620, doi:10.1002/14651858.CD003620.pub3.
184. L Abenavoli and S Bellentani, 'Milk thistle to treat non-alcoholic fatty liver disease: dream or reality?', *Expert Review of Gastroenterology & Hepatology*, 2013, 7(8):677–679, doi:10.1586/17474124.2013.842893.
185. S Zhong, Y Fan, Q Yan et al., 'The therapeutic effect of silymarin in the treatment of nonalcoholic fatty disease: a meta-analysis (PRISMA) of randomized control trials', *Medicine*, 2017, 96(49):e9061, doi:10.1097/MD.0000000000009061.
186. KM Gores, TS Hamieh and GA Schmidt, 'Survival following investigational treatment of amanita mushroom poisoning: thistle or shamrock?', *Chest*, 2014, 146(4):e126–e129, doi:10.1378/chest.13-1573.
187. DM Roberts, MJ Hall, MM Falkland et al., 'Amanita phalloides poisoning and treatment with silibinin in the Australian Capital Territory and New South Wales', *The Medical Journal of Australia*, 2013, 198(1):43–47, doi:10.5694/mja12.11180.
188. S Chuengsamarn, S Rattanamongkolgul, B Phonrat et al., 'Reduction of atherogenic risk in patients with type 2 diabetes by curcuminoid extract: a randomized controlled trial', *The Journal of Nutritional Biochemistry*, 2014, 25(2):144–150, doi:10.1016/j.jnutbio.2013.09.013.
189. L Vera-Ramirez, P Perez-Lopez, A Varela-Lopez et al., 'Curcumin and liver disease', *BioFactors*, 2013, 39(1):88–100, doi:10.1002/biof.1057.
190. RI Kashkooli, SS Najafi, F Sharif et al., 'The effect of berberis vulgaris extract on transaminase activities in non-alcoholic Fatty liver disease', *Hepatitis Monthly*, 2015, 15(2):e25067, doi:10.5812/hepatmon.25067.
191. R Huber, M Muller, J Naumann et al., 'Artichoke leave extract for chronic hepatitis C – a pilot study, *Phytomedicine: International Journal of Phytotherapy and Phytopharmacology*, 2009, 16(9):801–804, doi:10.1016/j.phymed.2009.03.007.
192. HF Chiu, TY Chen, YT Tzeng et al., 'Improvement of liver function in humans using a mixture of schisandra fruit extract and sesamin', *Phytotherapy Research*, 2013, 27(3):368–373, doi:10.1002/ptr.4702.
193. MA Leo and CS Lieber, 'Alcohol, vitamin A, and beta-carotene: adverse interactions, including hepatotoxicity and carcinogenicity', *The American Journal of Clinical Nutrition*, 1999, 69(6):1071–1085, doi:10.1093/ajcn/69.6.1071.
194. A Sheth, R Khurana and V Khurana, 'Potential liver damage associated with over-the-counter vitamin supplements', *Journal of the American Dietetic Association*, 2008, 108(9):1536–1537, doi:10.1016/j.jada.2008.06.443.
195. JN Hathcock, DG Hattan, MY Jenkins et al., 'Evaluation of vitamin A toxicity', *The American Journal of Clinical Nutrition*, 1990, 52(2):183–202, doi:10.1093/ ajcn/52.2.183.

196. D Carrington-Smith, 'Mawson and Mertz: a re-evaluation of their ill-fated mapping journey during the 1911–1914 Australasian Antarctic Expedition', *The Medical Journal of Australia*, 2005, 183(11):638–641, doi:10.5694/j.1326-5377.2005.tb00064.x.

197. D Shearman, 'Vitamin A and Sir Douglas Mawson', *British Medical Journal*, 1978, 1(6108):283–285, doi:10.1136/bmj.1.6108.283.

198. MA Farhangi, SA Keshavarz, M Eshraghian et al., 'Vitamin A supplementation, serum lipids, liver enzymes and C-reactive protein concentrations in obese women of reproductive age', *Annals of Clinical Biochemistry*, 2013, 50(Pt 1):25–30, doi:10.1258/acb.2012.012096.

199. DH Ipsen, P Tveden-Nyborg and J Lykkesfeldt, 'Does vitamin C deficiency promote fatty liver disease development?', *Nutrients*, 2014, 6(12):5473–5499, doi:10.3390/nu6125473.

200. W Zhang, XO Shu, H Li et al., 'Vitamin intake and liver cancer risk: a report from two cohort studies in China', *Journal of the National Cancer Institute*, 2012, 104(15):1173–1181, doi:10.1093/jnci/djs277.

201. S Gorman, LJ Black, M Feelisch et al., 'Can skin exposure to sunlight prevent liver inflammation?', *Nutrients*, 2015, 7(5):3219–3239, doi:10.3390/nu7053219.

202. RM Daly, C Gagnon, ZX Lu et al., 'Prevalence of vitamin D deficiency and its determinants in Australian adults aged 25 years and older: a national, population-based study', *Clinical Endocrinology*, 2012, 77(1):26–35, doi:10.1111/j.1365-2265.2011.04320.x.

203. R Chowdhury, S Kunutsor, A Vitezova et al., 'Vitamin D and risk of cause specific death: systematic review and meta-analysis of observational cohort and randomised intervention studies', *BMJ*, 2014, 348:g1903, doi:10.1136/bmj.g1903.

204. AJ Sanyal, N Chalasani, KV Kowdley et al., 'Pioglitazone, vitamin E, or placebo for nonalcoholic steatohepatitis', *The New England Journal of Medicine*, 2010, 362(18): 1675–1685, doi:10.1056/NEJMoa0907929.

205. SM Lippman, EA Klein, PJ Goodman et al., 'Effect of selenium and vitamin E on risk of prostate cancer and other cancers: the Selenium and Vitamin E Cancer Prevention Trial (SELECT)', *JAMA*, 2009, 301(1):39–51, doi:10.1001/ jama.2008.864.

206. ES Ford, UA Ajani and AH Mokdad, 'Brief communication: the prevalence of high intake of vitamin E from the use of supplements among U.S. adults', *Annals of Internal Medicine*, 2005, 143(2):116–120, doi:10.7326/0003-4819-143-2-200507190-00010.

207. Office of Dietary Supplements, *Vitamin E: fact sheet for health professionals*, National Institutes of Health website, 2019, accessed 1 August 2019, <https://ods.od.nih. gov/ factsheets/VitaminE-HealthProfessional/>.

208. G Bjelakovic, D Nikolova, LL Gluud et al., 'Mortality in randomized trials of antioxidant supplements for primary and secondary prevention: systematic review and meta-analysis', *JAMA*, 2007, 297(8):842–857, doi:10.1001/jama.297.8.842.

209. DE St-Jules, CA Watters, EM Brunt et al., 'Estimation of fish and omega-3 fatty acid intake in pediatric nonalcoholic fatty liver disease', *Journal of Pediatric Gastroenterology and Nutrition*, 2013, 57(5):627–633, doi:10.1097/ MPG.0b013e3182a1df77.

210. M Capanni, F Calella, MR Biagini et al., 'Prolonged n-3 polyunsaturated fatty acid supplementation ameliorates hepatic steatosis in patients with non-alcoholic fatty liver disease: a pilot study', *Alimentary Pharmacology and Therapeutics*, 2006, 23(8):1143–1151, doi:10.1111/j.1365-2036.2006.02885.x.

211. N Tanaka, K Sano, A Horiuchi et al., 'Highly purified eicosapentaenoic acid treatment improves nonalcoholic steatohepatitis', *Journal of Clinical Gastroenterology*, 2008, 42(4): 413–418, doi:10.1097/MCG.0b013e31815591aa.

212. HM Parker, JS Cohn, HT O'Connor et al., 'Effect of fish oil supplementation on hepatic and visceral fat in overweight men: a randomized controlled trial', *Nutrients*, 11(2):475, doi:10.3390/nu11020475.

213. R Aller, DA De Luis, O Izaola et al., 'Effect of a probiotic on liver aminotransferases in nonalcoholic fatty liver disease patients: a double blind randomized clinical trial', *European Review for Medical and Pharmacological Sciences*, 2011, 15(9):1090–1095.
214. A Alisi, G Bedogni, G Baviera et al., 'Randomised clinical trial: the beneficial effects of VSL#3 in obese children with non-alcoholic steatohepatitis', *Alimentary Pharmacology and Therapeutics*, 2014, 39(11):1276–1285, doi:10.1111/apt.12758.
215. J Sun and N Buys, 'Effects of probiotics consumption on lowering lipids and CVD risk factors: a systematic review and meta-analysis of randomized controlled trials', *Annals of Medicine*, 2015, 47(6):430–440, doi:10.3109/07853890.2015.1071872.
216. S Lontos, RM Jones, PW Angus et al., 'Acute liver failure associated with the use of herbal preparations containing black cohosh', *The Medical Journal of Australia*, 2003, 179(7): 390–391, doi:10.5694/j.1326-5377.2003.tb05606.x.
217. PJ Gow, NJ Connelly, RL Hill et al., 'Fatal fulminant hepatic failure induced by a natural therapy containing kava', *The Medical Journal of Australia*, 2003, 178(9):442–443, doi:10.5694/j.1326-5377.2003.tb05286.x.
218. H Helajarvi, K Pahkala, OJ Heinonen et al., 'Television viewing and fatty liver in early midlife. The cardiovascular risk in Young Finns Study', *Annals of Medicine*, 2015, 47(6): 519–526, doi:10.3109/07853890.2015.1077989.
219. S Ryu, Y Chang, HS Jung et al., 'Relationship of sitting time and physical activity with non-alcoholic fatty liver disease', *Journal of Hepatology*, 2015, 63(5):1229– 1237, doi:10.1016/j.jhep.2015.07.010.
220. M Palmer and F Schaffner, 'Effect of weight reduction on hepatic abnormalities in overweight patients', *Gastroenterology*, 1990, 99(5):1408–1413, doi:10.1016/0016-5085(90)91169-7.
221. K Purcell, P Sumithran, LA Prendergast et al., 'The effect of rate of weight loss on long-term weight management: a randomised controlled trial', *The Lancet: Diabetes & Endocrinology*, 2014, 2(12):954–962, doi:10.1016/S2213-8587(14)70200-1.
222. S Gleeson, 'A weighty issue for general practitioners: "Almario v Varipatis" (No. 2) [2012] NSWSC 1578', *Precedent*, 2014, 121:48–50.
223. JA Babraj, NBJ Vollaard, C Keast et al., 'Extremely short duration high intensity interval training substantially improves insulin action in young healthy males', *BMC Endocrine Disorders*, 2009, 9(3):1472–6823, doi:10.1186/1472-6823-9-3.
224. SE Keating, DA Hackett, HM Parker et al., 'Effect of aerobic exercise training dose on liver fat and visceral adiposity', *Journal of Hepatology*, 2015, 63(1):174–182, doi:10.1016/j.jhep.2015.02.022.
225. S Cheng, J Ge, C Zhao et al., 'Effect of aerobic exercise and diet on liver fat in pre-diabetic patients with non-alcoholic-fatty-liver-disease: a randomized controlled trial', *Scientific Reports*, 2017, 7(1):15952, doi:10.1038/s41598-017-16159-x.
226. CJ Lavie, JH O'Keefe and RE Sallis, 'Exercise and the heart – the harm of too little and too much', *Current Sports Medicine Reports*, 2015, 14(2):104–109, doi:10.1249/JSR.0000000000000134.
227. S Hayasaka, Y Shibata, S Ishikawa et al., 'Physical activity and all-cause mortality in Japan: the Jichi Medical School (JMS) Cohort Study', *Journal of Epidemiology*, 2009, 19(1):24–27, doi:10.2188/jea.je20080043.
228. T Dobzhansky, 'Nothing in biology makes sense except in the light of evolution', *The American Biology Teacher*, 1973, 35(3):125–129, doi:10.2307/4444260.
229. S Montagnese, B Middleton, AR Mani et al., 'Sleep and circadian abnormalities in patients with cirrhosis: features of delayed sleep phase syndrome?', *Metabolic Brain Disease*, 2009, 24(3):427–439, doi:10.1007/s11011-009-9146-5.
230. H Reinke and G Asher, 'Circadian clock control of liver metabolic functions', *Gastroenterology*, 2016, 150(3):574–580, doi:10.1053/j.gastro.2015.11.043.

231. K Chin, T Nakamura, K Takahashi et al., 'Effects of obstructive sleep apnea syndrome on serum aminotransferase levels in obese patients', *The American Journal of Medicine*, 2003, 114(5):370–376, doi:10.1016/S0002-9343(02)01570-X.
232. CW Kim, KE Yun, HS Jung et al., 'Sleep duration and quality in relation to non-alcoholic fatty liver disease in middle-aged workers and their spouses', *Journal of Hepatology*, 2013, 59(2):351–357, doi:10.1016/j.jhep.2013.03.035.
233. K Wijarnpreecha, C Thongprayoon, P Panjawatanan et al., 'Short sleep duration and risk of nonalcoholic fatty liver disease: a systematic review and meta-analysis', *Journal of Gastroenterology and Hepatology*, 2016, 31(11):1802–1807, doi:10.1111/ jgh.13391.
234. MH Jarrar, A Baranova, R Collantes et al., 'Adipokines and cytokines in non-alcoholic fatty liver disease', *Alimentary Pharmacology and Therapeutics*, 2008, 27(5):412–421, doi:10.1111/ j.1365-2036.2007.03586.x.
235. K Spiegel, R Leproult, M L'hermite-Baleriaux et al., 'Leptin levels are dependent on sleep duration: relationships with sympathovagal balance, carbohydrate regulation, cortisol, and thyrotropin', *The Journal of Clinical Endocrinology & Metabolism*, 2004, 89(11):5762–5771, doi:10.1210/jc.2004-1003.
236. C Li, JJ Xing, AQ Shan et al., 'Increased risk of nonalcoholic fatty liver disease with occupational stress in Chinese policemen: a 4-year cohort study', *Medicine*, 2016, 95(46):e5359, doi:10.1097/MD.0000000000005359.
237. TC Russ, M Kivimaki, JR Morling et al., 'Association between psychological distress and liver disease mortality: a meta-analysis of individual study participants', *Gastroenterology*, 2015, 148(5):958–966, doi:10.1053/j.gastro.2015.02.004.
238. KP Wright Jr, AL Drake, DJ Frey et al., 'Influence of sleep deprivation and circadian misalignment on cortisol, inflammatory markers, and cytokine balance', *Brain, Behavior and Immunity*, 2015, 47, doi:10.1016/j/bbi.2015.01.004.
239. M Wolfram, S Bellingrath, N Feuerhahn et al., 'Cortisol responses to naturalistic and laboratory stress in student teachers: comparison with a non-stress control day', *Stress & Health*, 2013, 29(2):143–149, doi:10.1002/smi.2439.
240. M Carev, N Karanovic, J Bagatin et al., 'Blood pressure dipping and salivary cortisol as markers of fatigue and sleep deprivation in staff anesthesiologists', *Collegium Antropologicum*, 2011, 35(suppl 1):133–138.
241. L Papanastasiou, S Fountoulakis and IA Vatalas, 'Adrenal disorders and non-alcoholic fatty liver disease', *Minerva Endocrinologica*, 2017, 42(2):151–163, doi:10.23736/S0391-1977.16.02583-9.

Index